Intermittent Fasting: No Diets Involved

Susan Stewart

Intermittent Fasting success stories from women that have worked with Susan Stewart

Anne-Marie's Story

I have been part of a wonderful group lead by Susan Stewart for 1 year now. I wanted to share how beneficial it has been for me and how I recommend this group to anyone wanting to change their eating habits for health and mind. After having my son Fox, I had another deep vein thrombosis scare which luckily only ended up being my superficial veins. I am on a list (which is non-existent at the moment) to get a procedure on my leg but needed to know I was doing something to help in the meantime...

I contacted Susan and she gave me lots of helpful advice on fasting and how it could really help if not mend the problem! This information, along with the want to get to my ideal weight, made me join and I haven't looked back since

I am now 2 stone lighter and closer to my ideal weight which I know I am getting to without starving myself and jumping from diet to diet. I feel so much better knowing the good that I am doing for my body and who knows, when it comes to operation time, I might not even need it! Susan is so supportive and knowledgeable and is there to answer any question. There is also a lovely group of ladies who all have their advice and successes to share, and it is so inspiring and motivating to be part of such a wonderful group. Anyone who wants to improve their health, body and mindset, I 100% recommend reading this book

Juliette's Story

I am always in awe of Susan's insight as a health coach and entrepreneur. She has been guiding my Intermittent Fasting journey in such a wise, gentle, and yet powerfully effective way. It feels like a breeze to implement the changes she suggested based on what I shared about my lifestyle.

The support I have received is second to none. My favourite part is that Susan always oozes kindness and joy - filling my heart with confidence and ease. This is helpful when I hit the "brick wall" and need guidance in the most aligned direction.

Susan listens to my feedback and always helps adjust the course in a way that feels "correct" to me.

On a personal level, I have rarely met such a reliable and resilient to adversity person. Susan Stewart is an inspiration, and I feel honoured that our paths crossed in such a transformational way.

Words from those who have read the book

From the moment I opened this book, I felt like I was sitting in a room with a warm cuppa across from a wise friend who was sharing her story back into wellness. This book is very easy to read. I finished it in two evenings and I know it's a book I will come back to time and time again for its wisdom. It felt like a gentle and wise hand guiding me through a very welcomed and practical journey into a way of life that would benefit me greatly. Susan's knowledge is impeccable and continuously backed up with evidence that has you paying attention. If you are someone who has struggled or is struggling to maintain a healthy lifestyle beyond yo-yo dieting, this book is for you.

Genevieve McGuiness, leader of the SoulTribe Temple, the SHE Sacred Holy Embodiment, Sacred Heart Circles, and the Priestess Path of Remembrance Retreats

The information in this book is not intended to replace the advice of the reader's own doctor or other medical professional. You should consult a medical professional in matters relating to health, especially if you have existing medical conditions, and before starting, stopping, or changing the dose of any medication you are taking. Individual readers are solely responsible for their own health care decisions. The author and publisher do not accept responsibility for any adverse effects individuals may claim to experience, whether directly or indirectly, from the information contained in this book.

CONTENTS

This book is dedicated to my grandchildren, Jack, Mimi, Daniel and Evelyn. The realisation that I want to run with you, play with you and watch you grow up was the main instigator of my Intermittent Fasting lifestyle.

Acknowledgements

This book has been written from the deep need to share this beautiful lifestyle around the world. My mission in life is to enable as many people as I possibly can to embrace this Intermittent Fasting lifestyle and leave 'diets' behind, to enable them to live a long, healthy, energised life.

I have been able to impact people with the sharing of my health programs and I want to thank each and every person who has joined me and embraced this new lifestyle. You absolutely rock and there is nothing better for me than witnessing your transformations.

I would also like to thank Katie Oman for keeping me on track, editing and getting me to the point of publishing with such love, honesty and beauty. Eileen Macdonald for being my first set of eyes and giving me good, honest feedback. My daughter Aimee for supporting me on the writing of the book and being a great sounding board for ideas. Genevieve McGuiness for her inspiration, spiritual guidance and accountability partnering. Not ever forgetting my Grannies Bella and Mary who ate fresh and well and were always there for me in my life. Forever grateful to you all.

Introduction

I was born in 1960, in the Highlands of Scotland. During those times we ate fresh, whole foods as that was what was available to us. In our village we had a dairy farm (where I would go and pick up our fresh milk everyday), a beef farm (I was delighted when the farmer named a new calf after me – yes, there was a cow called Susan). We had a huge garden full of vegetables. My uncle would fish daily before we woke and one of my earliest memories at 5 years old was going out to the washing line first thing in the morning to help him clean his nets. Sometimes I wore my Mum's stilettoes…I was always a bit of a style icon, in my own small way.

Food was abundant, fresh, and most of the time delicious. Although I do remember my Granny boiling tripe, and I still to this day feel ill as I conjure up the memory of that smell – it was vile to me. Most foods in our household were amazing though. We were lucky during those times, healthy and blessed to have such delicious offerings. We had a plum tree that grew up the side of our house, strawberries, gooseberries, raspberries, peas in pods, tomatoes, potatoes, lettuce, and cucumbers. In fact, anything that could be grown, my

Grandad grew it and grew it well; his garden was his pride and joy.

So, what happened to the world? What has impacted us and our health, weight, and longevity? I hope to cover all of this in this book as well as introducing you to a new lifestyle of intermittent fasting with no diets involved.

One of the filters I use when deciding what to eat is asking myself *"Would Granny have eaten this?"* It's the best filter as both my Grannies were the wisest of women who knew what was good for them and us, and also knew that the odd sweetie did us no harm at all.

Through sharing my own journey of diets, slimming clubs and yo-yo dieting I hope you find familiarity and realise that simple changes can allow you to leave that lifestyle behind. I hope they offer you true freedom from diets and enable you to enjoy the very best of health, sustainable weight loss, natural happiness and love for your body for the rest of your life.

"It is simple and easy." So many people tell me after joining my programs. The main reason for writing this book is to

share with you the way I found is best for me and many others and to take the confusion out of Intermittent Fasting. I believe we do not need to diet, calorie count, do keto or anything else vaguely like this. Introducing Intermittent Fasting to your life in the way I share in this book, is a way that you will be able to continue forever. It really is a new way of life – no cliché's involved. It will become the way you want to continue living and it will fit it into your life, not the other way around. You can still enjoy sociable times, holidays, barbeques, and nights out with no guilt attached; in fact, you will enjoy them even more than before. You will start to absolutely LOVE food, enjoying every morsel and you naturally will make choices around what you eat that suit your body.

All of this is included in this little book. I want everyone to feel as good as I do and the hundreds of people I have already shared this process with do.

"Everyone should be fasting and why aren't they?" was the question that would swirl around my mind constantly. Why the whole world doesn't know about this lifestyle and how it impacts not only weight loss but health, wellbeing, energy and longevity. This book is my small way of spreading the word on how to become the very best version of you.

Chapter 1

The Realisation

As I lay on the sofa feeling the weight of life on my whole body, I thought to myself that there must be more to life than this. I had eaten a huge dinner which put me into a coma state. I had my usual chocolate and crisps on the table beside me for when I felt like eating them in the not-too-distant future. Rubbish TV was on, and I scrolled through social media.

This was my norm; this was my life. What had become of me? What did my future hold? I would get up every day, go into my gorgeous boutique, and work for the day serving women and helping them look their best with our beautiful clothes. I know I seemed vibrant but inside I wasn't. I was tired, overweight, and often ill. I had been diagnosed with arthritis too. I had no energy, brain fog and never went anywhere socially unless it was for business. This was my life.

As I scrolled through social media, I noticed someone talking about their BMI. I thought to myself that I had never checked mine, so in the boredom of my evening, I went onto the NHS website which would tell me where I was on the BMI scale. I knew I wouldn't be healthy, but I really didn't expect the result that came up – Morbidly Obesc! Who? Me? I sat up in shock. I knew I was overweight but not to that extent. I redid the test putting in my height, weight, age, activity levels.

Morbidly Obese- what the hell did that mean? I read that I was at great risk of developing type 2 diabetes, heart problems, breathing problems, inflammatory diseases etc. No wonder I had arthritis. The site then went on to tell me to measure my waist as this is a good way to check you're not carrying too much fat around your stomach, which can increase your risk of heart disease and stroke. Yes, it was far too high a measurement. I was killing myself slowly but surely. This was my true rock bottom.

When did this start, I wondered to myself? I thought back to when I was 37- 20 years previously. I had gone from a size 10 to a size 12 and this was the first time I joined a slimming club. I didn't have much to lose, but I got sucked into the 'age, menopause' thing and thought I would get a grip of myself before weight started creeping on. Little did I know that these very slimming clubs would lead me from being a size 12 to a size 22 some 20 years later.

I was successful- hurrah! I went back down to a size 10, reached my target with ease, was awarded my certificate, and when off on my merry way feeling fabulous. Unfortunately, it didn't take long for me to gain the weight I had lost and then some. This time I was up to a size 14! Normal and healthy eating didn't make a difference. I had been on a low-fat diet at a slimming club (which I later found out meant high sugar). As soon as I added in fats again (even healthy ones), the weight came back on and more. These diets weren't sustainable, but I didn't realise that then. If only I had known that these slimming clubs rely on 84% of us failing and 74% of those individuals coming back and starting again. This is good as a business model for them because if we all succeeded and the weight stayed off, they wouldn't have a business. Looking back, it is obvious but at the time I was sucked into their propaganda, and I thought it was me that was the failure.

Fast forward 20 years and 40 diets later- yes, I tried them all. I was 6 sizes larger, which is 12 unhealthy inches around my waist alone and 55lbs heavier than when I started 'dieting'. Every time I went back on a 'diet' I would be a few pounds heavier than the last time I started. This was the pattern of my late 30's, 40's and 50's. Dieting made me gain weight and I now know that this is the norm for most women.

Thinking back, I do wonder if the diets were fully to blame, for I had a challenging life. Things happened in my childhood that I hadn't dealt with, which impacted me into adulthood. Feelings of abandonment, abuse, and feeling different were all parts of my story. I was a pretty woman, but sometimes attracted the wrong kind of person when all I was looking for was love. Very often, this led to disastrous results and heart-breaking endings.

In a way, I didn't really notice the weight going on. I would sometimes be walking past a shop and see myself in a window, and at first, not realise it was me! Was the weight creating a safety barrier for me? No longer being or feeling attractive was my way of keeping myself safe from heartache.

By the time I was in my 40's I was no longer interested in any kind of romantic relationships, so maybe I was making sure that they didn't happen by being less attractive than I used to be. *After all, who would want me now? Look at the size of me; I had let myself go.* I used to think things like this all the time. Now I know that I was keeping myself safe, instead of really dealing with my life and my ability to love.

In my early 50's I entered Cognitive Behavioural Therapy, which helped me deal with my life as it was. It was 6 months of deep work, every single day. I couldn't work during it, thankfully, I was on sick leave, and it was funded privately by my employer. I was lucky to be able to access it. I had to face my life head on and embed this into my life in a way that was manageable. I was given coping mechanisms and it worked. I had hit my rock bottom mentally and at last was doing something about it.

Now I was at my physical rock bottom. Whatever caused it, I now chose to take responsibility for my physical life. I had been researching Intermittent Fasting (IF) for around 3 years. I had several American friends who had great success with IF, but they included diets alongside it- KETO, low fat, and calorie counting. I knew this wasn't for me as it would just be another diet. The more I studied it the more I realised that if done gently with 'clean fasting' then hopefully it would work; no diets involved. I wanted to wake my body up and listen to what it told me.

So, I got up from the sofa, wrote my plan, and started right away with a bottle of water in my hand. I had a schedule which would give me fasted times and eating times. Nothing else was needed: no fancy foods, no counting calories, and no 'cheating days' (there is no such things as cheating and guilt). All I really needed was hours in the day, water and food. I was done with dieting. This really was the start of a new way of life for me and I was more than READY for it!

I was amazed at how easy it was! My biggest challenge was no cream (and I took a huge dollop) in my coffee in the mornings. It took 3 days for me to start enjoying black coffee and I still love it (you feel quite classy asking for a black coffee in a café). It took around a week to stop feeling hunger and I never again stopped at the convenience store on the way home for a family bar of chocolate and a tub of Pringles crisps- yes, I used to eat that nearly every single night.

Within 6 weeks I felt my energy rise, and I mean it shot through the roof! I loved that feeling, it was like, *"Oh my goodness, there I am! There's Susan! This is who I am- where have I been?"* I would never lie down of the sofa, and I hardly ever watched TV; I had too much to do, and I had the energy to do it. I hadn't felt like this since before I had children nearly 40 years ago! I would have to force myself to go to bed at night as I really didn't feel tired!

Within 2 months, the joint pain that used to cripple me had gone. The arthritis that my doctor had diagnosed me with a year before and told me would get steadily worse as it was just my age was leaving me! And I meant it completely left me- I never now suffer arthritic pain. Yes, it is a miracle.

My brain fog, which really did worry me, disappeared! I started remembering everyone's names, and I stopped forgetting what I went upstairs for. I was able to have wonderful conversations without searching for words that wouldn't come and forgetting what I was talking about. I would spend time on self-development, learning new things, and embracing new schools of thought on everything. My brain was on fire, fully alert. I had no more forgetful episodes and I was ready to learn and absorb everything again!

I felt happy most of the time, too. One of the beautiful effects of IF is that when we go into ketosis, as well as burning fat and glycogen, we also release a neurochemical called gaba into our brain, which in turn floods our bodies with dopamine and serotonin. This naturally enables us to deal with stress, anxiety, and even depression. I could handle stress and anxiety now. Most things just float over me, and if there was something I had to deal with, I deal with it from a place of peace.

One year later, I had lost 55lbs so easily, slowly and sustainably. I went from a size 22 to a size 12. I didn't exercise at all during my first year, but I felt as fit as a fiddle. I could run after my grandchildren. I developed many new interests, and I had the energy to fully immerse myself in them. It felt like I had gained so much more time in my life, but it was the increased energy and self-belief that I had that were the game changers for me.

I had 3 holidays that year and didn't fast fully throughout them. I mean, if someone is cooking you breakfast and I have paid for it, I will have it…some days. The first thing I would do as soon as I reached the airport on my way home was get my fasting schedule going, get my water intake up, and any weight I had put on would quickly drop off- most of it would be inflammation and water retention. It is important to be able to add fasting into your life. It really is a lifestyle, and we need to be able to live our life and not view our lifestyle as restrictive.

With any previous 'diet' I had been on, I would have come back from holiday feeling like a failure. I'd blown it, so what the hell- I'm just going to eat everything. This never happens with IF, for once it's embedded into your life, it will be there forever.

So, what about the food I ate? The most wonderful thing happens with IF- after your first few weeks, when your body is going through its healing stage, you go into appetite correction. You hear what your body is telling you. You no longer rely on outside signals like calories, points or syns to decide what to eat. Your body is intelligent, but we have just forgotten or been conditioned to not listen to it. You will be given signals when you have had enough to eat. That feeling of a food coma after eating isn't 'normal' as I used to think; it is your body telling you something you ate doesn't suit you. You naturally eliminate foods that make you feel like that, and these are different for everyone.

Foods that leave you feeling bloated are also telling you that they are wrong for you. Once you start realising this, you naturally veer towards beautiful nutritious foods without anyone having to tell you what to eat. You are intelligent and your body is too; it talks to you. I try not to eat normal dried pasta as it makes me sleepy, but fresh pasta is fine. That tells me that it's the chemicals that are used to dry or preserve pasta that don't agree with me. Bread is another no go for me. It bloats me. However, I have found Polish bread is fine for me as it doesn't have the sugar and chemicals that we put in so much of our British bread. It's wonderful to get to know your own biochemistry and what foods actually feed you well.

Then there's sugar! As time has gone one, I have found the dangers of refined sugar in my everyday 'diet' can creep in and sabotage me. I will cover this later in detail in the book. A little of what you fancy does you no harm, and the wonderful thing is you will no longer need or want to eat a whole cake or a complete packet of biscuits (like I used to). I used to say that I didn't eat a lot! I was lying! I now make the best choices I can. I eat healthy, nutritious food probably 90% of the time, and now and again I will have a cake or my favourite cheesecake. I eat it mindfully, enjoying every morsel, and I absolutely love every bite with no guilt attached.

I reckon that if two out of ten occasions when we are tempted to have a sugary 'treat' we succumb, then so be it. It is so important though to eat mindfully. When I decide to have a dairy chocolate or a bag of sweets, I always eat it slowly, and ask myself- is this as delicious as I thought it would be? More often than not, it tastes too sweet or even of chemicals, and the 'treat' is put down. I eat a lot less of it than I would have done in the past, so even that 2/10 times succumbing turns out to be so much less often than I would have eaten before. I did exactly this with a bag of Munchies yesterday. They were in my shopping basket before I thought about it and in the car, I opened them. I was so disappointed; they tasted awful. I was trying to remember what they had tasted like in the past and they definitely didn't taste of chemicals like they do now. My palate has changed and it's saving my life. A great tip for you is not to go grocery shopping when you are hungry as often these 'treats' jump out at you and your willpower will be at its lowest.

The beauty of intermittent fasting is that food starts to taste SOOO good! If it doesn't taste good, it's not suited to you. I began to love food more than ever before- actually love, celebrate and enjoy it. I eat slowly now, savouring every mouthful. I used to be the first one finished at every meal, but now I am the last as I take my time to enjoy every morsel. This happens naturally. I've probably become a bit of a 'food snob' as it's important to me to eat food I enjoy and that gives me all of the nutrients that my body needs. I'm delaying my eating times and not grazing all day long, as I see my choices as something to enjoy. The same will happen for you. I eat as 'clean' as I can most of the time. By that I mean I enjoy choosing organic or farm bought rather than supermarket foods. I trust our local farmer a lot more than I trust any supermarket with my nourishment.

I'm not saying that the journey to my new way of life hasn't been without challenges. There were still times when emotions would try and take over and I would find myself in the fridge or cupboard looking for something to satisfy my sadness or anxiety. Sometimes I didn't notice right away what I was doing, but the beauty is that I would realise after a few mouthfuls that I was trying to eat or suppress my emotions, and I would stop and say to myself, *"No Susan, this isn't you, this is the old you. You don't need this, phone someone, have a dance around the sitting room, or go out for a walk."* Most of all I would ask myself what the problem was and what I needed to know to help me with it. It worked every time.

Chapter 2

Starting Life Begins Intermittent Fasting Programs

My working life was mainly in the corporate world and media, and I had some really exciting jobs during my career. I worked for the BBC as a researcher and freelance interviewer when we still cut and spliced tape. I could take a breath out of a recording with a scalpel. Then along came digital technology, which was something amazing to learn to do, a whole new concept.

I worked in telecoms during their digital revolution. I can remember telling clients about voice over internet protocols, and that they would soon be able to speak to people through their computers not down telephone lines. It took a lot of explaining and look at us now – it's the norm.

I ended my corporate life working for BSkyB, having started as a business coach and ending up representing Sky retail on the marketeer's floor. This entailed flying to London on the red eye every Monday morning and returning on a Thursday evening. I stayed in beautiful hotels during the week with gorgeous restaurants- all on my expense account. I found it virtually impossible to maintain a healthy lifestyle during these times. I wish I knew then what I know now about fasting – it would have worked perfectly!!

I took early retirement when I was 53 as I had been ill with labyrinthitis. I got so dizzy that I couldn't function, I couldn't drive, I couldn't look at a computer screen or a television; a darkened room was the safest place for me. It also led to a very dark time in my life. When you can do nothing but lie down in darkness, your whole life comes back to you and there were many things that I had repressed when I was living my busy life.

Now in my 50's, I realised it was the time to deal with them. When I got a bit better and was able to stand and function a bit more, I decided to go for CBT therapy – mentioned earlier in chapter 1. I was lucky that I had BUPA healthcare through my work, and this was a deep time of healing for me. It took months, but I was able to view my life and all that had happened in it honestly and with clarity- it really was life changing.

During this time, I made the decision that I wasn't going to return to my corporate life; I was going to take early retirement. I still couldn't drive and was pretty much housebound as the dizziness was still happening and I would never know when it would come on.

I decided to fill up some of my time by going through all my clothes and selling all the corporate wear. It was cathartic and it also meant that I really wouldn't go back to my corporate life and job. It also helped me start planning for my future.

I sold my clothes on eBay and made a sizeable sum. My sister asked me to sell hers and a few friends then also asked me to help them selling their clothes, so that's what I spent my time doing. It got a bit overwhelming though as instead of clearing space in my home, I was filling it again with other peoples' clothes when I was photographing and selling them for them!

I did realise that there was something here in what I was doing, for every woman I knew had far too many clothes. Many of them absolutely gorgeous, but they didn't want them anymore, and someone else would love them. They were too good/valuable to donate to charity and there was a small fortune in their closets! I could help them with that.

Within a couple of months, I found premises in the town centre, converted it and opened a boutique. Amazingly, my labyrinthitis left me, I wonder if it was the Universe was saying slow down, you're home! It is time!

It was a fun experience and helped the environment, for it stopped clothes going to landfill and made it acceptable to wear second hand clothes – we called them preloved. I would only accept clothes that were good brands or designer, and women loved the shop. At first, they wouldn't tell their friends that they bought them from the boutique, but eventually I would see events being photographed in local publications and women proudly saying they had purchased from us.

I also visited schools educating children on the harm that fast fashion was doing to our world. Learning that fast fashion was the second biggest polluter in the world really hit home to these young people. We launched an upcycling competition where the children would make an outfit from something that they may have thrown away and it got a wonderful response. Some children showed real talent and were clothes designers in the making. One day a woman came into my store and said that her son had been in awe of my presentation, and I had changed the way he thought about clothes, and she thanked me for it – my job was done!

All in all, it was a rewarding experience. Another rewarding part of the boutique for me, was building women's confidence and showing them how to look at their whole selves in the mirror instead of focusing in on the parts of their bodies that they didn't like. We women are so hard on ourselves, and even to this day I encourage women to look at their whole self. You never walk into a room and people think, "*Oh, look at her belly*", they see the whole of you, from the inside out. I encourage women to look in the mirror daily and find things they love about themselves. To thank their bodes for the wonderful legs and feet that carry us around the world without thinking; their arms which carry easily and cuddle with love; and their heart that is so powerful and sends blood flowing around their body, as well as the deeper function of enabling them to love. The list is endless; our bodies need celebrating not shaming.

It was during this time that I had gone through my transformational journey through intermittent fasting.

Many women that came into the store would notice the difference in me and ask what I was doing, complimenting me on how well I looked. I would explain my version of intermittent fasting to them and so many of them would start their own journey with my guidance. I was helping customers, friends and family with their IF journey and it was working for them. I even typed up PDF leaflets that I would give out to them with step-by-step instructions.

My "*Aha*" moment came one day when I realised that I had more women come through the boutique door for advice on Intermittent Fasting than to buy clothes. I was handing out advice I had printed for women, and they were transforming in front of my eyes. Losing weight, becoming healthy, looking younger.

At the time I was taking business coaching from a wonderful woman called Darrell Sutherland. The coaching was for the boutique, as we were floundering at that point. We had enjoyed 4 good profitable years, won awards for being enterprising and the People's Choice Town Centre business, but Brexit was looming, and people had stopped spending money so freely.

On my next call with her, I mentioned that most days were being taken up handing out advice on intermittent fasting. She helped me see that I had a business right there that could be launched online, and I should stop giving away valuable advice for free.

Four weeks later, Life Begins Intermittent Fasting programs was launched, as an online 12-month program. I aimed to have 12 clients and I found them within days; all this as the pandemic started. During the next two years, I successfully launched one-to-one coaching for women who were more private and didn't want to be part of a group. That summer I also launched my membership: a program that was more affordable and that hundreds of women have gone through with amazing success.

My business continues to build and grow organically. I've now helped thousands of women from all over the world, from Scotland to Australia and back. There's nothing more inspiring than seeing them change their lives, ditch diets forever and transform their lives.

Yes, you can take the advice and guidance in this book and run with it on your own. I often give away my advice freely on social media, however, some women need extra help, guidance, and accountability. When working with me, we go deeper and it's nice to have someone to hold your hand and guide you through your life change

Chapter 3

Embedding Life Begins Fasting into my Life

At the time of writing this book, it is now five years since I started fasting, and it is my way of life forever. My health is amazing. I never get ill like I used to when I picked up every bug going and felt exhausted 90% of the time

The days of me avoiding social events as I was too tired, anxious or embarrassed are long gone. I can keep up with my grandchildren, play the games they want to play and not sit them out as Granny's legs don't work properly. What a thing to say to my grandchildren! I can now keep up with them, have the best of times and I'm not exhausted when they go home

The freedom this lifestyle has given me is immense and I know I am doing the very best for me. My longevity, my brain power, my bones, my everything! It's an amazing feeling knowing that I am in complete control of my future.

I no longer think about the hours I fast; I rely on my body telling me when I am hungry and when I am satisfied. I can distinguish hunger signals and real satiety – having enough to eat – signals. They were always there, I had simply given control away to outside signals, calories, diets, sugar cravings and the like.

I no longer wonder whether I have drunk enough water for the day during my fast. Water is now my drink of choice, and I know I will drink more than enough for my body to function properly. When I think of all those years, I never actually drank water, I wonder how I survived and didn't become seriously ill! I genuinely believe that if people simply started drinking 3 litres of water a day, they would cure many of their ills. We as a society are severely dehydrated.

In my first year of fasting, when I lost 55lbs, I didn't do any significant exercise. I concentrated on getting my fasting schedule embedded into my life and enjoyed the benefits. After this, I started three times a week doing a short High Intensity Interval Training workout in the morning. This entailed of 80 seconds of exercise and 20 seconds rest for a 15-minute workout. This is easily achievable and there are thousands of HIIT workouts on YouTube to suit people of all abilities. I would never feel like doing this but always felt elated afterwards. The beauty of this training is that it ramps up all the goodness that is happening during your fast by up to 40%. I now recommend this to women who are on my programs and the difference in weight loss between those who do and those who don't is significant. I can think of Lorraine who lost 5 stones in a year – this was due to her adding in early morning exercise to enhance the benefits of her fasted time. Try this simple tip put 2 grains of pink Himalayan salt under your tongue before the exercise, as well as making sure to hydrate during and afterwards.

I now love walking and walk 6k first thing in the morning every day, usually along the seashore (I am lucky to live 2 minutes from the Moray Coast in the beautiful Highlands of Scotland). I walk with my friend Nancy, so it's also great for my mental health as it means I gain connection for the day, great for your cortisol levels. We walk the same path each day but as it's beside the sea, every day is different. The sea can be calm or stormy, and some days we see the mountains in the distance, some days they are covered by cloud.

If you had said to me 5 years ago, that I would love walking I would have said, *"I can hardly walk up the stairs!"* I love walking so much that my friend Nancy and I, as well as two of my cousins are walking the Camino de Santiago later this year: 500 kilometres from France to the south of Spain through the Pyrenees. Yes, life really does begin at whatever age you realise life is for living!

I have enjoyed several holidays, social events, barbeques and parties over the years since I started fasting, and I have loved every single one of them. Sometimes I close my window and fast, sometimes I carry on and eat drink and be merry. The choice is mine, but at no point do I ever feel that I've "fallen of the wagon", blown it or failed in any way. I now love the fact that I have had a sociable time and been able to celebrate with no guilt. Yes, freedom is a wonderful thing.

I didn't lose any more weight after year one as my body decided that this weight and size is right for me, but body re-composition did happen. My waist got smaller, my boobs lifted (yes miracles do happen!) my skin got progressively better, lines disappeared, and even a long-term scar that I had for 40 years, which used to be quite red and unsightly, disappeared.

I had also been dealing with internal scarring – adhesions that were attached to the inside of my body from an operation that I had when I was 19. These used to cause me discomfort and doctors said that nothing could be done for them. They must have improved, as I never experience the pain that I used to from regular flare ups.

Occasionally, I will gain a little bit of weight. This usually happens when I'm on holiday and stop listening to my body or when I try to fit in with other people's schedules, but generally it drops off quickly once I get back to my fasting schedule and routine. It is often water retention, which I can feel through inflammation in my body as it reacts to being out of fasting schedule.

One tip I would give you that I did all through lockdown and still do now, because I have got so used to wearing leisure clothes most of the time, is to wear jeans one day a week. It will keep you in touch with your body weight and your comfort. For me, I love being able to wear jeans again after all those years of not being able to. In fact, my main motivator during my first year was a pair of size 12 bootcut jeans that I bought when I started and hung outside my wardrobe. It took me ten months to get into them and that felt so good!

In general, I am in what you call 'maintenance' mode. Your body decides the best weight for you, and you will stop losing weight at that point. As much as in my head I would love to be a size 8/10, I know that for my body, that isn't the right size. I continue to fast for as long as I did when I was losing weight – some days longer – but my body knows that it doesn't have to lose weight anymore.

My body does however still go through the beautiful health benefits every day and keeps me well, cleansed, rejuvenated and the very best version of me that I can be.

Chapter 4

Introducing Intermittent Fasting to your life – Choosing your Schedule

It is important to fit Intermittent Fasting into your life and not your life into Intermittent Fasting.

I advise starting very gently – many people are tempted to dive straight in at 18 hours fasted and go through the *no pain no gain* philosophy. I would advise you against this approach. Those days are long gone. We are introducing a new lifestyle. Intermittent Fasting – the "Life Begins "way is best done gradually, and the most important thing to do in the first few weeks is start with a shorter fast and make sure you get your water intake levels right.

Work out what is important to you. If it's sitting down and having dinner with your family, then prioritise or schedule your family meal at the end of your eating window. (We talk about fasting window and eating window). For example, if you have family dinner at 6.30pm, start your fast when your dinner is over- that could be around 7.30pm.

I have known some women who like to open their eating window in the morning as breakfast is more important to them. Tailor your fasting to fit in with your life, remembering that as you progress, your eating window will become shorter.

I recommend starting fasting for 14 hours fasted and having a 10 hour eating window for week one. **During your fasting window** you have to drink at least 1.5 litres of water-

Week 1 – 14 hours fasted 10 hour eating window and 1.5 litres of water in fasting window

Week 2 - 15 hours fasted 9 hour eating window and 2 litres of water in fasting window

Week 3 – 16 hours fasted 8 hour eating window – same water as above

Week 4 – 17 hours fasted 7 hour eating window – 2.5 litres of water in fasted window

Week 5 – 18 hours fasted 6 hour eating window – same water as above.

It is important that this volume of **water is to be drunk in your fasted time** – this is your real key to success.

Some people, especially if you haven't been used to drinking water may find the water intake a challenge. Firstly, water is water, but it can be drunk in so many ways-

- Cold from the tap
- Filtered if you wish – there are some great filter jugs out there
- Iced water
- Room temperature water
- Boiled water
- Carbonated water – remember unflavoured.

My top tips for getting used to the amount of water you need to drink are

1. When you close your eating window drink half a litre in the first 20 minutes of your fast, then sip on water until an hour before you go to bed
2. Take half a litre of water to bed and leave it overnight to reach room temperature. Make it the first thing you

do on waking, and drink within the first few minutes of waking – it is so beneficial for your body to do this.

3. Drink the balance of what water is left before your eating window opens

4. Drink from something you enjoy drinking out of i.e., a favourite crystal glass or glass bottle. The research done on plastics for our health is damning so I advise to avoid plastics if at all possible

5. Drink at least 2 cups of boiled water a day – it speeds up your metabolism – I often drink boiled water after my 2 black coffees in the morning and after each meal

In no time at all drinking water will become second nature to you. Initially you will be visiting the loo more, even during the night, but this will slow down after the first couple of weeks. Always remember the beautiful health benefits that water is giving your body.

It is very important that you follow the guide below on what you can and can't have during your fasted time. Remember we are keeping your insulin levels low so that you enjoy all the beautiful effects of your fast, so please follow exactly as I advise to the letter. The minute you put milk in your coffee, lemon in your water, drink fruit, herbal or flavoured teas or taste a piece of the packed lunches you may be making for you children, your insulin rises, and you effectively break your fast.

It has got nothing to do with calories – it is all to do with flavours and flavours trigger a spike in your insulin level – which will take you out of your fast. So if you add lemon, fruit teas, milk, sweeteners or anything at all apart from what is on the list below then your fast is broken and your insulin rises. (There are many schools of thought on this, but I am sharing what has worked for me and the thousands of women I have worked with. I am sharing with you the Life Begins fasting protocol.)

If you feel hungry, shaky or nauseas during your fasted time, my best tip is to use pink Himalayan salt (buy organic for this as many of the pink salts available are dyed pink!) It is a natural mineral, and these symptoms can be caused by lack of electrolytes. Pink Himalayan salts have 6 of the electrolytes your body needs and just a couple of grains under your tongue and you will feel better within minutes. If you don't feel better after trying this, especially in your early weeks, stop your fast and eat something and start again with your normal schedule later that day. Pink Himalayan salt is also helpful if you don't like the taste of black coffee, I find a couple of grains will take the bitterness away.

What is allowed during Clean Fast

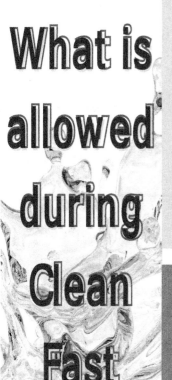

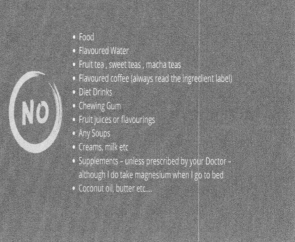

- Water, Sparkling water, soda water - all unflavoured
- Any plain tea with NO flavourings - black tea, green tea - tea bags are fine always check ingredients label as they can be deceiving
- Black Coffee (unflavoured) with caffeine, decaffeinated as above check the label for flavourings
- Mineral water
- Pink Himalayan Salt
- Electrolyte supplements (pure)
- Medications as prescribed by your doctor but always check if it is necessary to take them at specific times or can you take during your eating window?
- Peppermint Essential Oil for breath freshening only - I use WOW drops they can be bought on Amazon

YES

NO

- Food
- Flavoured Water
- Fruit tea , sweet teas , macha teas
- Flavoured coffee (always read the ingredient label)
- Diet Drinks
- Chewing Gum
- Fruit juices or flavourings
- Any Soups
- Creams, milk etc
- Supplements - unless prescribed by your Doctor - although I do take magnesium when I go to bed
- Coconut oil, butter etc....

THIS IS THE MOST IMPORTANT PART OF THE PROGRAMME.

WHEN YOU GET THE CLEAN FAST RIGHT YOUR BODY REPAIRS AND WILL BURN EXCESS STORED FAT

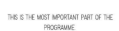

OK, I can hear you say – well, what do I eat? The honest truth is I am not going to tell you what to eat at this early stage, I will make some suggestions later in the book but for now your fasted time is the most important factor of the process. Remember your body is waking up. If this is your first delve into intermittent fasting, it may feel uncomfortable right now with me not giving you advice on food, however in a couple of weeks you will be messaging me and telling me that you understand why I haven't given you an eating plan! I want you to start listening to your body and hearing what it is telling you.

I would warn you to not take this eating window as your chance or opportunity to eat non-stop – that could be a hangover from previous unlimited foods diets. So, you eat 'what you like' means the food that you currently like. Listen to your body after eating – if a food makes you feel bad, tired, or bloated, cut it out but don't restrict yourself obsessively in the way you would with a 'diet'. Remember you will be eating a lot less anyways because of your fasted times. Your body will start waking up and your tastes will change naturally.

In the first few weeks of your fast the following happens –

You begin Intermittent Fasting with full glycogen (sugar) stores. You won't get into ketosis (fat burning) that day, or even necessarily for the first few weeks. Every day, you will deplete some of your glycogen stores. As you deplete more glycogen than your body adds back into storage during the eating window, you get closer to fat burning. (Not all of your food goes into glycogen storage after you eat.) Over time, you take out more glycogen each day than you put back in, and through the daily IF clean fasts, the amount of stored glycogen reduces.

After fasting clean for as long as it takes for you to deplete your glycogen stores sufficiently, the glycogen gets low enough that your body switches over to fat burning, and ketosis kicks in

Eventually, it may take days, or it may take a few weeks, you are at the point where you get into ketosis daily during the fast. I cannot say to you – you're a size 16 so that means it will take 6 weeks or you're a size 8 that will take 3 weeks. Everyone is different, so we just have to trust the process.

If you have underlying health issues it can often take a bit longer for ketosis to kick in and this is because of all the healing that is going on in your body.

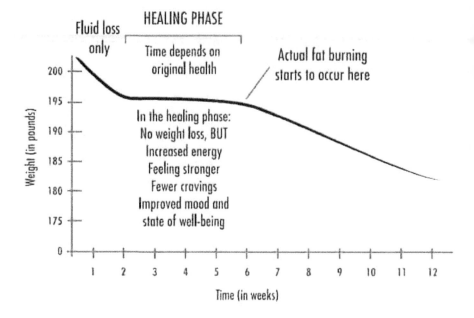

This diagram shows the process for some people. I always say weigh yourself on day one. I also recommend taking your measurements, taking photos of yourself in your underwear from the front, side and back, and taking a face selfie. After this is done, put the scales and measuring tape away for 4 weeks. The reason I suggest all 3 of these is that often with intermittent fasting we don't see the scale move but we lose inches and look different. The scale is not always a good guide, and we must also consider the way we are feeling as our body heals.

Some people lose weight in the first 4 weeks, some don't- but that is OK. This is a life change you are going through, and rest assured all the healing that is going on in your body is life changing in itself. I didn't lose any weight in my first 5 weeks, and it then took me a year to lose 55lbs. This was slow, healthy, sustainable weight loss and here I am 5 years later still maintaining, still feeling amazing and still living my life and enjoying food.

The first weeks are your foundational weeks, you are building the foundations of the rest of your life. You are getting used to fasting and your body is getting used to you treating it so well. It has probably taken you a good few years to reach the point of this life change, so please don't expect miracles and huge weight loss quickly. This is not a diet, and you won't be queuing to get weighed next week. We are on a different path to the very BEST version of you

I can't emphasise enough the importance of you drinking enough water during you fasted times as this will enable your body to go into flow and everything to work the way it's supposed to.

During the first 3 to 8 weeks, you go through the glycogen burn. All the glycogen and toxins will be leaving your body and then your body will become 'fat-adapted'. This is when you go into ketosis and start burning fat every single day.

How do you know you're in ketosis? First of all, your energy will rise. Maybe for a couple of days before your metabolic switch is turned on you may feel a bit tired and lethargic where the body is doing the final glycogen push and then – BOOM! Your energy is there, most times better than ever. You may also get a horrid taste in your mouth. Believe it or not, this is the fat burning, for we breathe 90% of it out in our breath. Your body odour may change and become stronger; again, this is the fat leaving your body. I use a good natural deodorant. The good news is these side effects settle down as time goes on, but you will continue to burn fat.

Your appetite will have started to correct, and you will soon start knowing when you've had enough to eat and when you are actually hungry. If you find that the new energy isn't coming by around week 6, then I would advise using a castor oil pack across your liver. This is made up from some muslin or even some old cut up towel, organic castor oil around 250mls. Heat it up (be very careful it doesn't get too hot), soak the cloth in the castor oil, and place across your liver (under your right breast and halfway across your left breast). Seal with some cling film, place a hot water bottle over the top and lie down for 2 hours!

Repeat this every week for 4 weeks (you can use the same pack simply keep it in an airtight container in the fridge it will keep for 4 weeks just heat it each time). The effect of this is that it will open up the bile ducts around your liver and encourage drainage which may have been slightly blocked.

The way fasting works is that your body will always burn glycogen first, which is the sugar that you have consumed. Hopefully you will have naturally reduced your refined sugar intake during your first few weeks. It also applies to alcohol, as its main ingredient is sugar. What I would advise is if you do drink alcohol keep to white spirits and avoid sugary mixers. I used to love a gin and tonic but the tonic (even Fever Tree botanical), believe it or not, started to taste far too sweet. Yes, I was upset! I now have soda water and a slice of lime or a bloody Mary with freshly squeezed tomato juice.

I don't drink alcohol as often as I used to. I have a new rule that I will drink on a social occasion, and I generally will only have a couple of drinks. They still have the alcohol effect, but I find that's enough for me these days. I drink them mindfully and enjoy every sip. They take ages to drink, and I love them, but I don't want to be the drunkest person at the party!

I would also advise limiting or choosing to drink alcohol to one day a week if you socialise and drink no more than a couple of drinks, if you can. The way I would look at it is that the next fast, where you will have inevitably closed you window later that day, will prioritise the glycogen burn and that is it. Be happy that you've had a great time! Open your eating window as normal the next day and that's you back to normal fasting schedule, safe in the knowledge that the alcohol and sugar is burnt away. You won't have undone all the good that has already happened in your body – it's just a day in your life. You are a faster now and your body knows it!

During the first 4 weeks approximately, there is amazing transformations going on in your body...

Detoxification Stage 1

On the first day of fasting, your blood sugar level drops. Your heart rate slows, and blood pressure is reduced. Glycogen is pulled from your muscles which could cause some weakness. The first wave of cleansing can be the worst. Headaches, dizziness, nausea, bad breath, and a heavily coated tongue are signs of the first stage of cleansing. Hunger can be the most intense in this period. My best tip for you is if you feel any of these effects (some people don't) is a couple of grains of organic pink Himalayan salt under your tongue or in your coffee will help. What you may be lacking is electrolyte balance and in this natural mineral you will gain 6 of the electrolytes your body needs

Detoxification Stage 2

Fats, composed of transformed fatty acids, are broken down to release glycerol from the glyceride molecules and are converted to glucose. The skin may become oily, as rancid oils can be purged from the body. People with problem-free skin may have a few days of pimples or even a boil. The body embraces the fast and the digestive system is able to take a much-needed rest, focusing all of its energies on cleansing and healing. White blood cell and immune system activity increases. You may feel pain in your lungs. The cleansing organs and the lungs are in the process of being repaired. The breath is still foul smelling, and your tongue may be coated. Within the intestine, the colon is being repaired and impacted faeces on the intestinal wall start to loosen. □

Detoxification Stage 3

You will experience enhanced energy, clear-mindedness and feel better. On the downside, old injuries may become irritated and painful. This is a result of our body's increased ability to heal during fasting. If you had broken your arm 10 years before, there is scar tissue around the break. At the time of the original break, the body's ability to heal was directly related to lifestyle. If you lived on a junk-food or unhealthy diet, the body's natural healing ability was compromised. During fasting, the body's healing process is at optimum efficiency. □

As the body scours for dead or damaged tissue, the lymphocytes enter the older, damaged tissue secreting substances to dissolve the damaged cells. These substances irritate the nerves in the surrounding region and cause a reoccurrence of aches from previously injured areas that may have disappeared years earlier. The pain is good as the body is completing the healing process. The muscles may become tight and sore due to toxin irritation. The legs can be worst affected, as toxins accumulate in the legs.

Detoxification Stage 4

The body is completely adapting to the fasting process. You will experience energy and clarity of mind. Cleansing periods can be short with many days of feeling good in between. There are days when the tongue is pink, and the breath is fresh. The healing work of the organs is being completed. After the detoxification mechanisms have removed the causative agent or render it harmless, the body works at maximum capacity in tissue proliferation to replace damaged tissue. After day 20, the mind is affected. Heightened clarity and emotional balance are often felt at this time. Your memory and concentration improve.

So, there you have it. There are amazing happenings going on right there inside your body and all this happens within the first approximately 30 days. It is mind blowing that this is going on inside your body.

Chapter 5

8 Weeks and Onwards

After your first few weeks, around 8 weeks in, you will no longer need to check the clock for opening your eating window. You will be able to start trusting yourself and knowing when you are hungry. You will generally be at 18 hours fasted with a 6-hour eating window (some days a bit more some days a bit less) and you will naturally be drinking the water that your body requires. Always let your thirst guide you. Some days you will feel like eating a lot, other days you won't be so hungry- listen to that.

Keep your body fed and energised with whatever you fancy to eat. Learning to honour our hunger and knowing when it is real hunger comes quite quickly in our Intermittent Fasting Program.

Now a little bit about food! I'm ready to talk about it!

I would suggest that you include protein when you open your eating window. A portion the size of your palm is enough. Do you know that if you ever feel hungry it is protein you are hungry for? Your body is never hungry for carbs, although we do need them. I always think it's good to get some good protein in right at the start of your eating window – probably 3 to 4 days a week, especially if I've had a day before where I didn't need much to eat. Fish or eggs are my go-to foods. Another tip is if you feel that maybe you haven't eaten enough in a day but are no longer hungry is to have a hard-boiled egg as you close you eating window; you won't then get hungry for protein later. I boil a dozen eggs and keep them in the fridge – they are safe for 7 days and I eat a lot of them. It is a myth that they are bad for your cholesterol. Probably another piece of research funded by the dreaded food industry.

For fruit, try to remember diversity is key for a wide range of fruits. Probably around 3 days a week I open my eating window with a nice big bowl of fruit - everything from banana, strawberries, raspberries, grapes, and sometimes some watermelon. It is good to eat fruit on an empty stomach, it is pre-digested and the cleverest of our foods. It is bright and tempting – who couldn't resist plucking a ripe orange from a tree or popping a deep red strawberry from a plant? It is clever because its seeds are non-digestible, so even although they bypass through our system they are designed for self-propagation.

Our DNA is linked back to times millenniums ago. We used to eat fruit in season at the end of the summer when it was ripe, and it would feed us up for the winter when food would be scarce. We would naturally live off our body fat stores. The sugar from the fruit would turn to fat cells – that's how sugar was naturally evolved to feed and nourish us. It also self-propagated so that there would be crops of it for next year.

For carbs, I stick to unrefined carbs as much as possible. Refined carbs spike your insulin and even although your insulin rises when you eat anything, if we can keep that spike lower most of the time, then less of what we eat is turned into fat cells and our body doesn't have to work so hard when we are fasting. I have to say I love potatoes though and will eat them with their skins on (great nutrition right there). I do this maybe 3 days a week generally with my meal as I close my eating window.

By unrefined carbs, I mean-

Unrefined whole grains –brown rice, barley, quinoa, oatmeal.

Non-starchy vegetables – spinach, green beans, Brussels sprouts, broccoli, celery, tomatoes.

Legumes – kidney beans, baked beans, peas, lentils.

Nuts – peanuts, cashews, walnuts.

Fruit – apples, berries, citrus fruit, bananas, pears.

Do I eat potatoes, turnip, and carrots? Yes, I do, just not every single day. General rule of thumb I have is that if it's grown above the ground have lots of it, below the ground in moderation.

Most breads are inflammatory and have chemicals and sugar included to preserve and to make us eat more. Do you know that many brown loaves are just white bread with caramel colouring! Bread really bloats me and does for many people; I also believe that people may think they are coeliac but actually it's just the chemicals added to the bread that they are not suited to.

Then there's fats. Don't be fearful of them! Fats in general aren't bad for you, in fact they are absolutely vital for your wellbeing and often aid absorption of vitamins to your body e.g., a drizzle of olive oil on your salad will give you more absorption of the vitamins from your salad vegetables.

Oils I use-

- Extra virgin olive oil for dressings and for medium heat cooking
- Avocado oil or coconut oil for high temperature cooking
- I use butter not margarine and Ghee which is even better

I avoid all other oils due to their toxic, carcinogenic, genetic modification qualities within them, and for my general health

We need Omega 3 and Omega 6 as they are anti-inflammatory and very important for our health. I would eat oily fish 3 times a week.

Omega 3 food – oily fish, nuts, eggs

Omega 6 foods – olive oil, avocado oil, ghee, seeds, avocados

What I would call a decent nutritious plate of food is a palm size portion of protein, a fist size portion of non-refined carbs, half a fist of starchy carbs if wanted and a good drizzle of oil, an avocado or the like.

When we combine protein with carbs, the effect of the carbs is totally different. Protein buffering happens, which in basic terms helps maintain a healthy PH balance in your body. Our insulin and blood sugars don't spike, and our body won't have to work so hard in our fasted time.

All in all, you will naturally be eating a lot healthier that you were prior to starting your new lifestyle. However, it is good to keep in mind the advantages of some food groups on our body.

Will your body adapt, and weight loss stop?

This is such an important point to understand. When you follow an intermittent fasting lifestyle using these strategies, you don't have to worry so much about your body adapting. If, however, you are a rigid with your mealtimes or are used to calorie counting, that may be a problem.

Here's why...

The body absolutely can adapt to anything you do that's the same day-in and day-out. If you eat the same exact number of calories, as an example, or always eat the same small meal in a 30-minute eating window, then yes, your body can adapt to that pattern. Your metabolic rate can adjust to match what you are eating, and your weight loss may come to a halt.

I am often asked- **does your body adapt to your eating plan and fasting lifestyle?**

The answer is yes. Sometimes it can, but here are some strategies that you can apply to stop your body from adapting to a specific level of caloric intake or rigidity of timings. And great news! If you are listening to your hunger and satiety signals, and adjusting your intake based on those signals, you are already on the right track.

I don't eat the same way every day, and I don't ever suggest that you should eat the same way every day, either. In fact, I say that you should learn to listen to your body and adjust intake as needed within your daily eating window.

Even though I generally eat within a 6-hour window, sometimes it's 4 hours, sometimes it's 8 hours. I rarely have 2 meals, instead I often have a snack or bowl of fruit to open my window, then a meal later, or vice versa. They're not ever the exact same amounts, the exact same length of time, nor are they the exact same nutrients and I have no idea the number of calories – they really are irrelevant. Whilst fasting, remember that we use stored calories and nutrition (which we use during our fasted time) as well as real time calories that we eat, and the nutritional value is a lot more important. Even the times that I open and close my fast change day by day. You can now trust yourself to really listen to your body, hunger, and satisfaction signals. Nothing is the same about it from day to day. Some days I will eat 2 meals if I'm hungry, on holiday I may even eat 3 meals.

It is important that you learn to listen to your body. Don't be overly rigid in your intermittent fasting lifestyle. Don't schedule a rigid window that is exactly the same every day. In fact, time in the end doesn't matter. You will be used to having a period of time that you fast, hydrate and let your body do the magic and a time that you eat and fuel your beautiful body; it will go along with your life and lifestyle.

You are now at the stage that you can trust your body to tell you when you're hungry. Don't count calories or have food that's exactly the same every day. i.e., don't open your eating window with the same sandwich every day, or have the same salad for dinner. Don't aim for some sort of dietary perfection. You can leave the 'diet' mindset behind you in your previous dieting life. You can now relax and enjoy life and love food more than ever.

You learn to-

- Be more flexible and fit fasting into your beautiful life.
- Listen to your body. It is intelligent and speaks to you and tells you what it needs.
- Eat more some days, eat less on other days. This happens naturally and hey, I still love a full Sunday roast with all the trimmings! But, when I do have this, on Monday I will eat very little. That's absolutely fine, in fact, your body and metabolism will enjoy the unpredictability of it.
- Vary your window length- go with the flow.
- Live your life.

One day your body may be satisfied with a very small amount of food. It's fine to stop eating and learn to trust those satiety signals. The next day you may need a longer window because you are hungrier, so eat more- that's fine too! Trust that your body needed more, rather than beating yourself up because you are a failure, fallen of the wagon, blown it or some such nonsense. Those days are over. Take a day off for a special occasion. Live a little when life allows.

This is not a diet; it's a lifestyle. As I have said before, your diet mindset will be the biggest hurdle for you to get past. Please understand this point: making the lifestyle rigid and diet-like is counter-productive to your goals and I want you to succeed and live your best life. It's both as simple and as complicated as that.

Will you plateau and stop losing weight?

Yes, this can happen, and for many reasons. It may be that you have become too rigid with your timings, eaten the same thing too often or sometimes your body has just got used to fasting and needs a bit of help to retrigger weight loss. As long as this isn't your final plateau, which is detailed below, these are the things I would advise you to try.

- Really mix up your fasting window. Have one day where you stretch yourself and have a short eating window – say 4 hours – but make sure you eat enough during that window. So, this is the one time I would say go past satiety, fill yourself up, and close your window with something high in good fats – avocado, peanut butter, olive oil dressing, or hard-boiled eggs. The next day see how long you can extend your fast to. An extra hour will make all the difference. Use pink Himalayan salt – a couple of grains to stave of hunger.

- For 3 days a week open your eating window with no carbs, eat vegetables that are grown above the ground, no sugars even hidden ones, and have your carbs later in the day. This will elongate your fast and fat burning and allow your insulin to rise slowly rather than spiking quickly.

- Try a Liver Cleanse – this is detailed at the back of the book, and I advise all my clients to do this once every 3 months to make sure our liver is working like the filter it is. Eat no processed foods for 5 days so it will stop your sugar cravings in their tracks.

- Do a food edit – really look at the foods you are eating, even keeping a diary and see if processed foods and refined sugars are prevalent in your diet. Even although we don't like the taste of them anymore, they can creep back into our eating and before we know it, we are hooked again. We can get a bit complacent with our eating as time goes on so it's good to revaluate from time to time

The wonderful final plateau will be when your body reaches the perfect size and weight for your unique biochemistry. By then you will be the absolute architect of your body and that is the best feeling in the world.

When you do reach "*your ideal weight*," your weight loss will stop. Who decides that you are now at your ideal weight? Surprise! It's not your conscious brain. It's your body. When your body decides you are at the ideal weight for you and your lifestyle, you will stop losing weight and you will be at a permanent plateau. Ideally, it will be at a weight that your conscious-self also thinks is your ideal weight. My body stopped losing weight when I reached around a size 12. I continue to fast in the same way as I always have, and I know my body is clever enough to know what's 'right' for the unique me!

Remember: if you enjoy this lifestyle, then relax and enjoy the journey. You won't lose all of the excess weight quickly. I lost on average 1lb a week in my first year, but that mounted up to 55lbs! You may get to a point, like I have, and stay at approximately the same size, with a very gradual loss of extra fat over time. Eventually, you should get closer and closer to your ideal weight, and your body will decide when you are there. Not you. It may be higher or lower than you thought it would be, but rest assured it will be perfect for **YOU.**

Chapter 6

Emotional Eating

Give Yourself Kindness Instead of Food

Anxiety, loneliness, boredom, anger and pain are emotions that we all experience throughout our lives. Each has its own trigger, and each has its own solution or appeasement.

Food doesn't fix any of these feelings, although we may find short-term comfort in opening the cupboard and grabbing the crisps, chocolate, cheese or wine. It will never satisfy the void we are feeling in the long-term and can often make us feel worse. Try and identify your triggers and stop there. Consider a solution, whether it be phoning a friend, a walk-in nature, three deep breaths, or a glass of water.

Ultimately, you will have to deal with the source of the emotion, which takes time and depth of feeling.

Do you know that feeling? Your emotions take over and the next thing you know, you are in the cupboard looking for something to make you feel better. Before you know it, you've gone through the whole cupboard, the fridge, eaten everything and you still feel awful. In fact, you feel worse because that horrid guilt kicks in on top of your emotional turmoil.

We treat food as our friend to fill the void of

- Loneliness
- Depression
- Sadness
- Grief
- Stress
- Anxiety
- Pain

It can be our crutch when we think that we have no other option. I've been there many times, having that food is your friend feeling.

The thing is that food will never solve our problems, never has and never will. WE create these habits that don't serve us, and we feel trapped when the answers are often so simple.

Admitting we are lonely is a big step – it is viewed as a failure in many societies – but it is only a feeling and there will be friends or even a specific friend that you can contact and chat this through with. Even if it's a passing feeling, I know if someone I knew contacted me and asked me for a chat because they were feeling lonely, I would say of course. It's often something within us that feels vulnerable and shameful to admit loneliness. So, the next time you feel lonely, leave the cupboard closed and think to yourself – who could I call that would listen? You will have someone.

Depression is an absolute trigger for going to the cupboard and the fridge. *"I'll eat this, and it will make me feel better"*. As I've already said, it won't, it will simply compound your issues and your feelings, make you feel like a failure and fill you full of guilt. Depression is a complex issue and there are so many things you can try. Firstly, when you make the decision to go to the cupboard to make you feel better, just stop right there, check in with how you are feeling at that point, wait for 5 minutes – even just 1 minute the first time. Often the fact that you have made a decision to address your feelings is enough and exactly the right time to sit with it and ask yourself, *"What do I need to know to help me feel better?"* It's worth a try. Also be sure to seek out professional medical support if you feel as though you are suffering from depression. There isn't a one size fits all fix for mental health, and there is no shame in reaching out for help.

Sadness comes from somewhere, but how often do we allow ourselves to simply sit and work out what is making us sad? Sometimes we just have to go there. Something I recommend is to get my journal out and write *What is making me sad?* and see what comes. Journal on it in as much detail as possible. Then read it back and from there list your problems. Next to each one (there may only be one) write a solution, give it a timescale for resolving if possible and you will feel amazing after.

Stress and anxiety – I am grouping these together as they are similar and often lead people to eating when they don't need to. My best advice is to totally divert yourself when feelings of stress or anxiety take over. Do things like put your favourite music on and dance, or go outside, even just in your garden, in your bare feet. Feel the ground underneath your feet and imagine you have roots going all the way down to the centre of the earth. Go out for a walk- I love walking by the sea, but just simple outside air and daylight will help. How beautiful is it to walk and look up and see the stars? It helps you realise how vast this universe is and how wonderful life is.

The very best cure for all of the above is Intermittent Fasting. In the past 5 years I have only had 3 occasions where I went to the cupboard and started eating my emotions. The beautiful thing is I realised what I was doing a few mouthfuls in and stopped, without anyone telling me or feeling guilty, bloated and a failure. It is so powerful realising that you are in complete control of your body; it is true body freedom.

Many women I have worked with have said the same and their biggest worry when joining me was that they were emotional eaters. When we listen to our body, we honour it and manage to leave these habits behind us. We reclaim our body as ours and the freedom that offers is truly liberating.

I have to talk about cortisol – the stress hormone – also known as our fight or flight hormone. This was so helpful to us when there were lions and tigers outside our caves but it's not so relevant to our lives now. Yes, of course we need to be aware when we are in danger, but realistically that mainly means stopping and crossing the road safety or not risking walking home by ourselves late at night.

Unfortunately, high cortisol levels can hamper our wellbeing. They can actually make you put on weight, not absorb nutrients that you eat and sabotage your fast if you are a faster. Cortisol is naturally highest first thing in the morning when we wake, so what I advise you to do is get control of them right there and then.

How I do this is to enjoy a 5/10-minute morning gratitude meditation before I get out of bed. There are thousands of meditations on Insight Timer: a wonderful FREE app. If I don't have time for this I will consciously rise from bed and, as I put my feet on the floor one foot at a time, I say thank you Goddess, God or Universe (use whatever is relevant to you) for a brand-new day. Then I have a big stretch. When I am brushing my teeth, I look myself in my left eye and inside my head I say I love you 10 times. When I started doing this, that little eye used to shed tears. It's now part of my routine and I feel the love in my heart... from me!

Then I get in the shower, and I look at my day ahead- from going downstairs and having my first wonderful coffee; to everything that is in my diary that I have planned for the day through to family dinner; a nice evening; and then off to bed again. I give everything the very best outcome, even if it's something I am not keen to be doing. The beauty is if everything goes wrong – I have already seen the best outcome and will veer towards it. It's called segment intention and I honour Abraham Hicks with this beautiful practise.

Prior to me finding this practise, I would very often naturally go through the day ahead in the shower and step out of it with dread. I now step out of it feeling happy and looking forward to the day ahead. And... my cortisol levels will be low.

Always remember you are the purveyor of your own happiness. Sometimes that can feel harsh, but if you are unhappy then you are allowing something or someone to make you that way. As always, you are in control.

Chapter 7

The Food and Diet Industry

I will start with the food industry...

Let's go way back to the 1960's- 1967 to be precise. Newly released historical documents show that a study was done by some Harvard scientists, who the sugar industry paid to play down the link between sugar and heart disease, instead seeking to promote saturated fat as the culprit.

The internal sugar industry documents, recently discovered by a researcher at the University of California, San Francisco, suggest that five decades of research into the role of nutrition and heart disease, including many of today's dietary recommendations, may have been largely shaped by the sugar industry.

"They were able to derail the discussion about sugar for decades," said Stanton Glantz, a professor of medicine at U.C.S.F. and an author of the JAMA Internal Medicine paper.

The documents show that a trade group called the Sugar Research Foundation, known today as the Sugar Association, paid three Harvard scientists the equivalent of about $50,000 in today's money to publish a 1967 review of research on sugar, fat and heart disease. The studies used in the review were handpicked by the sugar group, and the article, which was published in the prestigious *New England Journal of Medicine,* minimised the link between sugar and heart health, as well as casting aspersions on the role of saturated fat.

Even though the influence-peddling revealed in the documents dates back nearly 50 years, more recent reports show that the food industry has continued to influence nutrition science.

Last year, an article in *The New York Times* revealed that Coca-Cola, the world's largest producer of sugary beverages, had provided millions of dollars in funding to researchers who sought to play down the link between sugary drinks and obesity. In June, it was reported that sweetie makers were funding studies that claimed that children who eat sweeties tend to weigh less than those who do not. How ludicrous is that?!

The first study, which I view as completely corrupt, had a horrific effect on our health. Before 1970 there was no such thing as type 2 diabetes, it literally didn't exist. But, after this wrong information, people started eating sugary products. New products were also introduced: jars of sauces, processed and preprepared meals to name a few were becoming available and being labelled as 'healthy'. Our highly processed convenience foods started and took over, and they were all laced with sugar, not because it would enhance the flavour or for nutritional value but because it would make you eat more food. Eating foods containing sugar makes you eat more foods containing sugar. The OBESISTY epidemic was starting, and type 2 diabetes was born.

The figures for type 2 diabetes in the UK at the time of writing is more than 4.9 million people in the UK have diabetes, and 13.6 million people are now at increased risk of type 2 diabetes in the UK. Approximately 850,000 people are currently living with type 2 diabetes but are yet to be diagnosed.

It is important to remember that diabetes is not a death sentence. Research worldwide has consistently shown that, for some people, combined lifestyle interventions - including how and when you eat your foods, physical activity and sustained weight loss - can be effective in reducing the risk of type 2 diabetes by about 50%. The great news is that Intermittent Fasting may be able to reverse type 2 diabetes, and every woman that has joined my programs who has had type 2 diabetes and embraced my way of intermittent fasting has either reversed it or had a radical health improvement, so there is hope

The thing about sugar though is that it's as addictive as drugs. A review published in the *British Journal of Sports Medicine* has claimed that refined sugar has a similar effect on the brain as illegal drugs, such as cocaine.

In studies on rats, it has been found that there are significant similarities between eating sugar and drug-like effects such as binging, craving, tolerance, withdrawal, dependence and reward.

The research scientists claim that sugar alters mood and can induce reward and pleasure, in the same way drugs such as cocaine affects the brain. They cite studies in rats where sugar was preferred to cocaine, and studies in mice where the mice experienced sugar withdrawal symptoms. How scary is that? It is, however, true.

I am not saying to eradicate sugar from your diet completely. There are lots of ways of eating our sweet treats without eating foods laced with refined sugars. One of my favourites is dates and peanut butter, which is delicious, but buy organic dates, as if not they can be coated in glucose. I found this out to my dismay when I bought some recently at a well-known supermarket. Please buy wholefood organic peanut or cashew butter. If not, you will find sugar and palm oil is standard in peanut butter. 70% or above cacao chocolate is divine, you can't eat a lot of it, it is good for our cortisol levels (stress hormone) and even feeds our gut microbiome. I love the fact I have found a chocolate that is good for you! Another tip is: if you are craving sweet things, have a couple of olives as they neutralise your need for sugar. On the whole, Intermittent Fasting will refine your tastebuds and correct your appetite, and you will find that food that contain refined sugars or any of their derivatives will be too sweet for you and you will naturally not like them anymore

74% of processed foods contain some kind of sugar. Even a cooked chicken that I recently nearly bought, the third listed ingredient was brown sugar!

So, all I am saying here is to please be careful. If we can eat as healthily as we can, it will help our wellbeing and longevity. I'm not saying never eat sugar- I'm saying be aware. Let's not allow the food industry to corrupt us. We need take back control of what we eat.

Our bodies aren't designed to eat the way that we eat nowadays- to have breakfast as soon as we rise, graze until lunch, have lunch, graze until dinner then graze until bedtime. Our DNA is linked straight back to the caveman who ate by feast or famine. Our bodies can't cope with eating all day and night long; we're just not made that way! We end up ill and diseased. Our bodies aren't designed to eat sugar in the way it's processed today. Be very careful.

Then we have the chemicals that enter our food chain...and not in a good way! Humans have made, found or used over 50 million unique chemicals over the past 5 decades, and approximately 10 million of them have entered our food chain in one way or another. This can be pesticides on our crops and earth, chemicals fed to animals, drugs, hormones, antibiotics and other chemicals that are even fed to the animals we eat. There are also chemicals put in our food that turn off our leptin hormone which tells us we are satisfied in terms of how much we have eaten. There are also chemicals that turn on our ghrelin hormone that tells us that we are hungry. Yes, this is how corrupt the food industry and our governments are for allowing this to happen and

I am only touching on a small amount of corruption here. Research it for yourself to appreciate the full extent of the situation; there is a whole volume of books to be written on this subject.

If you can take back control and eat as much fresh and non-processed food as you can then you're on the right track for your health, wellbeing and longevity.

Let's look at our diet industry. How may actual 'diets' have you been on? I had tried them all…

The Cambridge Diet

Slimming World

Weight Watchers

The Cabbage Soup Diet (yes really!)

Calorie counting

Scottish Slimmers

The Mediterranean Diet

Atkins

Keto

Carnivore

Lighter Life

Paleo

To name a few!!

Did they work? Yes, most of them did in the short-term, but every single time I was successful I would go back to eating 'normally' and put all the weight back on that I had lost and more. So steadily over 20 years I slowly went up 6 dress sizes and gained 60lbs. Dieting made me morbidly obese!

I recently found an article that gave me the statistics I had been looking for. I wanted to know what percentage of slimming club members were successful and maintained their weight loss up to 2 years after they hit target weight. You would think they would have this information readily available as the slimming clubs must have this information... it took me years to find it.

The article was in a Sunday magazine, I think in the *Mail on Sunday,* and they had interviewed a previous financial director of Weight Watchers UK. He said that 16% of club members who hit target weight maintained this for 2 years or over, 84% failed and put weight back on, and 76% of those returned to the slimming club. He stated that this is 'good business". It proved my suspicions that slimming clubs rely on us failing- that's where they make their money! We have been duped! Again!

Further research told me that slimming clubs and diet brands use language in their literature; language to veer us towards thinking we are failures and to feel guilty! How dare they!

Detox

This is mostly a marketing language, and there's little consistency in what products mean when they make claims about removing "toxins" from the body. Besides, the liver and kidneys manage to effectively detox most people's bodies., especially if you are a faster.

Superfoods or Miracle Foods

While it's true that humans thrive when eating a balanced diet that's high in fruit and vegetables, most foods touted as super, or miracle are simply ... food. Many expensive and rare fad ingredients are the same as the produce on sale at your local supermarket.

Foods that are bad, toxic or poison

Some foods are not healthy when eaten in disproportionately large quantities, or to people with specific allergies, but the fear mongering language of referring to particular nutrients as "poison" or "toxic" is incorrect and counterproductive. Again, unless it's truly poisonous, it's probably just food.

Cheat Day

The concept of a "cheat day" comes from diet culture. For example, the way Weight Watchers encourages participants to take occasional days off from the program, or not count points for events like birthday celebrations. It's also an (unproven) weight-loss strategy that claims to reset the metabolism and make a very restrictive diet easier to follow. The language assumes everyone is dieting and suggests that restrictive eating is normal and a "cheat day" where you eat what you feel like eating is the exception.

Wellness

Sometimes it's just a nice way to talk about getting a massage or going to yoga; other times it's a way of re-packaging the diet culture into a friendlier seeming, but still highly profitable, business. The "wellness" industry has managed to market the thin, white, able-bodied ideal as a health concern rather than an arbitrary and class-based standard. True wellness is much broader than simply nutrition and exercise. The wellness wheel concept is a useful way to think about what else it includes. I use this wheel every 3 months to see where I need to do better.

"You look great! Have you lost weight?"

This common piece of body shaming small talk efficiently conveys that you think a person should be trying to lose weight. This is especially awkward if the person hasn't lost weight or has lost weight for a less-than-cheerful reason, such as depression, an eating disorder, or an illness. As a general rule of thumb, it's not polite to comment on the shape of people's bodies. I remember when I was losing weight people saying to me, "*Oh, don't lose any more weight*" – I always thought to myself, *why not?* I wouldn't say anything though.

The body you want; a perfect body; beach body

These euphemisms rudely assume every person is trying to get thinner. Not everyone is trying to lose weight. And, as food writer Mark Bittman and doctor David L. Katz recently wrote: *"Not everything that causes weight loss or apparent metabolic improvement in the short term is a good idea. Cholera, for instance, causes weight, blood sugar, and blood lipids to come down—that doesn't mean you want it."*

Atone or do Penance with Exercise

When we consider foods bad or sinful, it's natural to think that there should be a penance to pay for eating them, and exercise is often framed as the way to exact that punishment. This approach isn't the best way to sustain a healthy level of movement in daily life. Instead, consider what forms of movement and exercise make you feel great while you're in the act of doing them.

Earn Certain Foods

This is a kind of pre-atonement, suggesting that you must punish yourself with exercise to justify enjoying food. This message is not because the food is delicious and nutritious or your body is craving its nutrients, but because you earned it.

"I'm just concerned about your health"

'Concern trolling' can manifest as over-emphasising or invasively inquiring about health metrics such as weight or cholesterol levels, and it can be a way to fat-shame while maintaining a false veneer of polite concern.

War on Obesity or Obesity Crisis

The writer Michael Hobbes laid out brilliantly in the Huffington Post's Highline, where he spoke of how weight is an imperfect indicator of health. Any talk of the so-called scourge of obesity that does not acknowledge the systemic and societal factors that contribute to the condition's prevalence, and the ways that fat people are mistreated and misdiagnosed by the health care system, should be regarded with suspicion. Our industrial food system, a shame-based medical approach, and the stigmatising of fat people are all crises, too.

How would you feel if you never again have to 'diet'? If you can leave behind these diets that don't serve you, that will mess with your metabolism and your mind, and gain freedom from them forever! That is what Intermittent Fasting offers you. The freedom to trust yourself, to gain control of your own beautiful body and to finally find YOU inside who has been there all along!

Chapter 8

The Science of Intermittent Fasting

While fasting we are tapping into the endocrine (hormone) system, communicating between

- Body tissues
- Brain
- Organs
- Gland
- Muscles

This affects our

- Mood
- Digestion
- Stress level
- Sexual function
- Sleep
- Energy

- Blood sugar
- Ovulation
- Even fertility

Our hormones work as a team, these are:

- Oxytocin
- Cortisol
- Insulin
- Sex Hormones
- Progesterone
- Testosterone
- Oestrogen

While fasting, we repair cells to make them hormone sensitive again. This has the wonderful positive effects on our menstrual cycle, premenstrual syndrome, premenstrual tension, polycystic ovary syndrome and the menopause.

I have had many women freed from the drudgery of painful, irregular periods, night sweats from the menopause and many more hormonal challenges that us women face simply by introducing fasting to their lives.

I have also had the pleasure of being messaged by women who have fallen pregnant after introducing Intermittent Fasting to their lives and thinking that they couldn't have babies naturally. There really isn't anything that makes me happier!

We do this through the "Clean Fast"- that is only drinking water, black coffee, black or green tea with no sugars, milk or sweeteners, and no cucumber, lemon or fruits in our water. Our insulin stays low when we fast, and we go through the most incredible cleanse that has hourly benefits. It's all to do with insulin levels and the impact of flavours on them, and NOTHING to do with calories!

The Importance of Hydration During Intermittent Fasting

You most definitely will become dehydrated during intermittent fasting, if you don't follow the guidance on how much water to drink during your fasted time. This is partly because of the fact that around 20-30% of the water we get is from food and it comes mostly from fruits and vegetables.

But another major reason you may become dehydrated is due to the fact that, during fasting, your body will likely be flushing out a lot of water. This can even lead to electrolyte imbalance (which you can combat by simply adding a pinch of Himalayan salt to your water).

Some of the symptoms of dehydration during intermittent fasting can include fatigue, thirst, dry mouth, headaches, slow digestion, and bloating. So, make sure that you stay properly hydrated throughout the day. This will also help you to feel less hungry, especially when you are starting out with Intermittent Fasting.

Water is essential for keeping your body cells functioning. It also helps to boost the benefits of Intermittent Fasting. As the body enters maintenance mode, it starts to cleanse proteins and other structures that have died or become dysfunctional. Without enough water, the body cannot perform the necessary detox efficiently. This is why you need to take great care to drink plenty of water throughout the day.

The beauty of water fasting has so many benefits – including balancing your immune system and teaching your body's organs to absorb nutrients more effectively.

The hourly benefits of fasting are in my opinion and experience:

- Within 4-8 hours of fasting, blood sugars fall as all food has left the stomach
- In 12 hours, the food that had previously been consumed has been burned. The digestive system goes to sleep, body begins the healing process, and the human growth hormone begins to increase. Glycogen is relaxed in blood sugars
- In 14 hours, the body has converted to using stored fat as energy. Fat burning starts, and the human growth hormone begins to increase dramatically.
- 15 hours, autophagy starts where the body clears out damaged cells in order to regenerate new, healthier ones.
- 16 hours and over, the fat burning, autophagy, human growth hormone all ramp up

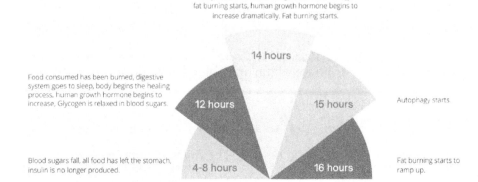

Body has converted to using stored fat as energy, fat burning starts, human growth hormone begins to increase dramatically. Fat burning starts.

14 hours

Food consumed has been burned, digestive system goes to sleep, body begins the healing process, human growth hormone begins to increase, Glycogen is relaxed in blood sugars.

12 hours

15 hours

Autophagy starts

Blood sugars fall, all food has left the stomach, insulin is no longer produced.

4-8 hours

16 hours

Fat burning starts to ramp up.

Intermittent Fasting boosts the human growth hormone (HGH) naturally by up to 3000% every day! In normal life we gain around 2-minute bursts of it a few times a day, with fasting we gain hours of it flowing through our body

Picture this: your body is healing itself with HGH every day, feeding your muscles, bones, aligning your metabolism, and turning on your anti-ageing genes. People pay substantial sums for HGH injections, when all they need to do is fast.

HGH also boosts muscle growth, strength, and exercise performance, while helping you recover from injury and disease

Human growth hormone is an important hormone produced by your pituitary gland. Also known as growth hormone (GH), it plays a key role in growth, body composition, cell repair, and metabolism.

Low Human Growth Hormone levels may decrease your quality of life, increase your risk of disease, and make you gain fat cells. Optimal levels are especially important during weight loss, injury recovery, and athletic injuries.

One of my favourite effects of Intermittent Fasting is Autophagy. This means getting rid of damaged and toxic cells and recycling them to new healthy ones.

In 2016, the Nobel Assembly at Karolinska Institute awarded the Nobel Prize in Physiology or Medicine to Yoshinori Ohsumi for his discovery of mechanisms for autophagy whilst fasting. Why is the world not shouting about this? Well, the pharmaceutical industries don't want us to be preventing illnesses or healing ourselves naturally. How much money would be lost to this multi-billion-pound industry?

But what is autophagy? The word derived from the Greek *auto* (self) and *phagein* (to eat). So, the word literally means to eat oneself. Essentially, this is the body's mechanism of getting rid of all the broken down, old cell machinery (organelles, proteins and cell membranes) when there's no longer enough energy to sustain it. It is a regulated, orderly process to degrade and recycle cellular components.

In simple terms it is cleansing and regenerating cells at the deepest level. It is our clever body's way of recycling our cells, getting rid of dangerous ones, rescuing and repurposing cells that can be saved, keeping us well and curing our ills

Who wouldn't want this to happen every day within their bodies?

Ketosis is the wonderful process of fat burning, and the great news is you don't need to do the Keto diet to hit fat burning. Intermittent Fasting triggers the exact same fat-burning process that occurs during a low-carbohydrate or keto diet, but we can still eat a nutritious diet. The great news is that you do not have to diet!! Keto is short for ketosis, the magical metabolic process that kicks in when your body runs out of glucose (its preferred energy source) and starts burning stored fat.

When we start our IF journey, your body will be going through many changes internally. It will also be getting rid of all the glycogen stored in your cells We get into ketosis when we deplete our glycogen stores sufficiently to switch over to fat burning.

As previously explained, it can take a while to reach fat adaptation and ketosis, and it is different for everyone with no real guidelines on how long it will take but when it hits you will feel amazing. Your energy levels rise, and you will start to lose weight slowly- around 1lb a week. However, that is sustainable, and rest assured your body is healing every day.

Add to that, ketosis also turns your happiness on! When we go into ketosis, which happens every day for established fasters, gaba is released to the brain which in turn floods our body with dopamine. This turns our happiness on and helps us deal with anxiety, depression, stress.

I know that my own stress levels and how I deal with stress has changed dramatically since I started fasting, and the women I work with tell me the same.

One woman in particular springs to mind. On a Zoom connection call in our membership, we were talking about this process as a group and she told us that her husband's nickname for her used to be 'Grumpy", and she said it was because she absolutely was grumpy. All the time she thought it was simply part of her personality, but 3 months into fasting he said to her, "*I can't call you grumpy anymore because you smile all the time!*" She said she had never felt so happy in her life and if this was the only thing that she benefited from with IF she would be eternally happy with that. She did also lose weight and gain the best of health

And.... during ketosis your cells are primed to stop viral replication, so we have at least 3 processes going on whilst fasting to keep us well.

Why doesn't everyone know this? We are cleansing our bodies, cleaning and regenerating our own cells, helping our bones, muscles, regulating our metabolism, and encouraging longevity. We are also losing weight, without any medication. Now there's the thing, in my opinion Big Pharma do not want us keeping ourselves healthy and curing our ills with something as simple as Intermittent Fasting.

Chapter 9

Fasting – the History and Spirituality

We have been fasting since time immemorial.

We are connecting into our bodies and waking them up, that in itself is a spiritual practice in my opinion. The answers to everything lies within us all. Why shouldn't our 'diet' and allowing our bodies to work the way they should be included?

Add to this the fact that it is encoded in our DNA. Think about it- before we had fridges, freezers, packaged foods and fast-food drive throughs, people naturally went long periods of time without food; our bodies encoded this into our DNA over millennia. It's important to think about the benefits of fasting from an ancestral and genetic perspective since we are all mostly working from the same DNA today, despite the fact that our lifestyles have changed dramatically, especially in the last 100 years. Researchers found that 99% of our genetics haven't changed in 10,000 years.

While our genes have remained relatively the same, our lifestyle has transitioned from hunting and gathering societies to farming cultures, which set off an era of food always being available. The water we drink, the air we breathe, the soil our food grows in, the food we eat and how often we eat it has changed dramatically in a very short period of time.

This has caused a mismatch in many ways. Fasting is encoded in our genes, but in general we don't do it. The fact that we don't has caused so many problems for-

- Health
- Wellbeing
- Weight
- Mental clarity
- Anxiety
- Body function
- Natural good health

Intermittent Fasting isn't something new, it is the way we are meant to **BE.**

Modern day breakfast was invented in 1908 by James Harvey Kellog with the strapline, *'Breakfast is the most important meal of the day'*. It truly isn't and that myth has been dispelled scientifically many times over. It doesn't speed up your metabolism, and it doesn't make you eat less during the day; it actually does the opposite. But what a clever marketeer Mr Kellog was, as I'm sure your Mum or your Granny would have told of breakfast's importance. It's simply another way the food industry has hoodwinked us.

Yes, we break our fast and always have done when we start to eat – but breakfast is not a necessary part of our eating regime.

Religious Fasting

Fasting is an important practice in many of the world's religions, carried out for a variety of reasons. A religious person may fast to cultivate personal discipline and spiritual energy, as a form of self-mortification, to commemorate special events, to follow tradition, or to symbolise and enact detachment from the world.

Bahá'í faith

Fasting is one of the greatest obligations of a Bahá'í. In the Baha'i Faith, fasting is observed from sunrise to sunset during the Bahá'í month of 'Ala' (between March 2 through March 20). It involves the complete abstention from both food and drink (as well as smoking). Observing the fast is an individual obligation and is binding on all Bahá'ís who have reached the age of maturity, which is 15 years of age.

Buddhism

Fasting is generally considered by Buddhists as a form of ascending and as such is rejected as a deviation from the Middle Way. Nevertheless, Theravada Buddhist monks and nuns, who follow the Vinaya monastic rules, traditionally do not eat each day after the noon meal. However, this is not considered a fast, but rather a disciplined regime for aiding in meditation.

The Vajrayana practice of Nyung Ne is based on the tantric practice of Chenrezig. It is said that Chenrezig appeared to Gelongma Palmo, an Indian nun who had contracted leprosy and was on the verge of death. Chenrezig taught the method of Nyung Ne in which one keeps the eight precepts on the first day, then refrains from both food and water on the second. This was seemingly against the Middle Way, this practice is to experience the negative karma of both oneself and all other sentient beings and, as such, is seen to be of benefit.

Christianity

Fasting is a practice in several Christian denominations and churches. Other Christian denominations do not practice it, seeing it as a merely external observance, but many individual believers choose to observe fasts at various times at their own behest. The Lent fast, observed in Anglicism and Catholicism, is a 40-day partial fast to commemorate the fast observed by Christ during his temptation in the desert. The Book of Isaiah chapter 58:3-7, discusses fasting saying it means to abstain from satisfying hunger or thirst, and any other lustful needs we may yearn for. The blessings gained from this are claimed to be substantial, patience, control and deepening of your faith. The opening chapter of the Book of Daniel verses 8-16, describes a partial fast and its effects on the health of its observers. Christ himself stated that certain blessings and healings would only happen with fasting and prayer.

In general fasting can be viewed as a spiritual practise – strengthening resolve, enhancing patience, enabling us to listen to our bodies.

Fasting is also arguably one of the oldest therapies in medicine.

Hippocrates believed it enabled the body to heal itself-
"…those desiring to lose weight, should perform hard work before food. Meals should be taken after exertion and while still panting from fatigue. They should, moreover, only eat once per day."
He also wrote:
"Everyone has a physician inside him or her; we just have to help it in its work. The natural healing force within each one of us is the greatest force in getting well. Our food should be our medicine. But to eat when you are sick is to feed your sickness."

Paracelsus wrote 5000 years ago that fasting is a great healing remedy
Ayurvedic medicine has for many centuries advocated fasting as a major treatment
Pythagoras was among many who extolled the virtues of fasting.

So, you see it's no new fad- it's part of our historic culture both spiritually and scientifically.

The healing traditions of fasting, ancient or modern, have one thing in common – they support the body to heal itself, rather than turning to medicines and physicians or to invasive treatment to treat illness or create positive change.

I have found that fasting has deepened my spiritual practise. Everything is about going within, and if our bodies are cleansed and working the way they should be then it translates through to our mind and our spiritual practises whatever your beliefs may be.

Chapter 10

The Freedom of Intermittent Fasting

The freedom that Intermittent Fasting the "Life Begins" way offers you is phenomenal and never ending. I myself have witnessed this as a serial yo-yo dieter of 20 years who had such guilt attached to "good" and "bad" foods. I used to talk about cheats, treats, rewards, syns and would constantly 'blow' a diet because I had had a holiday, a night out or just a cake. The freedom at the start was slightly uncomfortable. It can feel like a licence to eat.

When you have been brainwashed by the diet industry, the food industry and even your Granny who probably started the food reward thing. You know the one – you have fallen over, and you're given a sweetie to make you feel better, you get an ice cream as a 'treat'. The thing to remember though is that in Grannie's times there wasn't so many hidden sugars in our diets.

Getting past this is one of the biggest challenges to changing your lifestyle, as the diet mindset is engrained in our psyche. It was for me and for hundreds of women that I have worked with.

What if I tell you that food will no longer be your focus in life? You won't be spending hours of your week, planning meals, or thinking about what you will cook for dinner tomorrow. Yes, it's obsessive, isn't it? I can remember driving to work and that would be my main train of thought – what will I cook tomorrow, or the next day, or what will I have for lunch today?

The obsession goes and guess what? You start to love food. You will no longer be told what to eat. There are no meal plans to consider, no keto, no calorie counting, no points, no syns and no fads. You are the one that will listen to your body and hear what it wants to eat.

I buy lovely healthy nutritious foods that I love, like seafood, shellfish, organic meats, a diverse range of fresh vegetables and fruit (I have even started growing my own again), and nuts and seeds. I buy mainly wholefoods and as close to their natural source as possible. I very seldom plan ahead what I am going to eat, I know that the food I have in my fridge and my cupboards contain lovely, fresh and nutritious choices. I decide what I am having when I get hungry. You do become very choosy with your food as you have waited for it patiently and you feel that it has to be worth the wait.

We remove all the guilt that you attach to food...

- Food as a reward
- Food as a treat
- Going for a takeaway after slimming club (yes, we all did that)!
- I deserve this I've been good!
- Oh, I've blown this
- I've fallen off the wagon!
- Eating just in case you feel hungry later (yes me too!)

What wagon? There is no wagon to fall off. No guilt attached to it at all. No diet to be done, no calories to be counted and certainly no syns to be had!

Viewing food as 'Good or Bad'

Food is to be enjoyed-

- Our tastebuds wake up and food starts to start delicious
- We naturally reject foods that are full of sugar and chemicals because we no longer like the taste (yes miracles do happen!)
- We naturally eat more slowly
- We look forward to breaking our fast with something nutritious and really worth eating

Appetite Correction

We have 2 hormones in our body that tell us when we are hungry and when we are satisfied – Ghrelin and Leptin. Sadly, these have been turned off or at least, we aren't as aware of them as we could be because we have been relying on all these outside signals to tell us when to eat and what to eat. There are also chemicals and deadly fructose put into foods that turn these hormones off.

Then there is sugar...

There are currently at the time of typing this there are 64 different names and types of sugar in the UK. Here are the British Heart Foundation's 50 main ones:

https://www.bhf.org.uk/informationsupport/heart-matters-magazine/nutrition/sugar-salt-and-fat/names-for-sugar-infographic

5 0 SHADES OF SUGAR

You might see these on ingredient labels, but don't be fooled by their different names. They are all types of sugar, and too much added sugar is bad for your health.

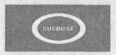

SUCROSE

DEXTROSE

BROWN SUGAR

SUCROSE SUCROSE

SUCROSE

BEET SUGAR

MALT SUGAR
MALT SUGAR
MALT SUGAR

MALTOSE

GOLDEN CASTER SUGAR

JAGGERY

ORGANIC SUGAR

DARK MUSCOVADO SUGAR

CRYSTALLISED FRUCTOSE

HONEY

FRUCTOSE

RAW SUGAR

🌢 AGAVE SYRUP
🌢 BARLEY MALT SYRUP
🌢 BROWN RICE SYRUP
🌢 CAROB SYRUP
🌢 CORN SYRUP
🌢 GOLDEN SYRUP
🌢 INVERT SYRUP
🌢 MALT SYRUP
🌢 MAPLE SYRUP
🌢 SORGHUM SYRUP
🌢 SUGAR BEET SYRUP

CORN SUGAR

CANE SUGAR

INVERT SUGAR

PALM SUGAR

COCONUT BLOSSOM NECTAR
COCONUT SUGAR

MOLASSES

CANE SUGAR
CANE JUICE

BLACKSTRAP
MOLASSES

DEHYDRATED CANE JUICE
EVAPORATED CANE JUICE

TREACLE

CARAMEL

MAPLE SUGAR

GLUCOSE
ISO GLUCOSE
GLUCOSE SYRUP
GLUCOSE FRUCTOSE
SYRUP

AGAVE NECTAR

SUGAR
SUGAR
SUGAR

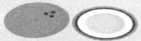

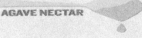
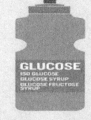

APPLE
JUICE
CONCENTRATE

FRUIT
JUICE
CONCENTRATE

GRAPE
SUGAR

DATE
SYRUP

DATE
SUGAR

All of these turn off your natural hormones which tell you when you are hungry and when you are satisfied, and they will make your body want more food within minutes of eating. There is a wonderful lecture done by the University of California - Robert H. Lustig, MD, UCSF Professor of Paediatrics in the Division of Endocrinology, explores the damage caused by sugary foods. He argues that fructose (too much) and fibre (not enough) appear to be cornerstones of the obesity epidemic through their effects on insulin.

Our bodies wake up with Intermittent Fasting. You will start to recognise when you are actually hungry and when you are satisfied. You will hear that ghrelin hormone and know it's hunger and the leptin hormone and know you are satisfied. Have you ever managed to feed a baby when they aren't hungry? Or keep feeding them when they've had enough? It is impossible to do because they are in touch with their hormones. Doesn't that tell you that this is learnt behaviour or a reaction to some kind of food additive and even conditioning by the media?

A little tip to know when you are satisfied when you start fasting- there will be a point during the meal that you take a big sigh (when I say this to my clients they often say, *"Oh that never happens to me"*. The next day they message me saying, *'You're right, I do sigh Susan!"*) This is your leptin hormone speaking to you – saying you've had enough. At that point, put your fork and knife down walk away from your food. Wait for 15 minutes and, if you actually feel hungry, finish your plate, but I am sure that won't happen. Another way to recognise you're satisfied is when your food stops tasting as delicious as it did when you first started eating it. This again is leptin saying – enough.

I am not saying to waste this beautiful food; put a cover over it and put it in the fridge. Nearly every day my next meal is made up from some of my last meal. It's great fun and you will feel so good and in control and you'll never have that feeling of being overfull again.

Several women have joined my programs and they were worried about their 'diet drinks' addiction. They were sure they would fail and would ask me, *"What can I do to stop it?"* I told every one of them not to worry about it, but to fast with the amount of water that they need to drink during their fasted time, and all will be well. They will naturally stop. Every one of them who took my advice stopped drinking diet drinks within days – 2 weeks at the most. They were amazed and so grateful.

The same thing happens with 'sugar addiction'- you will naturally stop liking the taste of refined sugars. I'm not saying you'll never have a chocolate bar again, but I am saying you will no longer be addicted to them. I used to eat a family bar of Galaxy at least 3 nights a week I wouldn't and couldn't even look at one now! Freedom!

You have to just listen to what your body is telling you. I never want to fall asleep after eating now as I know the foods that make me feel like that and I avoid them, in the same way as I avoid foods that bloat me. Life is so much better not going around half asleep or with a pregnant looking belly (at 61 it's not a good look). It's all so obvious but we have just forgotten to listen to our beautiful bodies.

Intermittent Fasting will wake you up to this. It makes you more aware, and you will start to listen and hear what your body is telling you. You will be energised, inflammation will go, you will feel amazing, and you will lose weight if you need to.

Chapter 11

The Microbiome: Gut Health

You know those sayings about gut feelings. Well, they're all true.

However, I want to talk to you about your beautiful gut and in particular your microbiome - the microorganisms in a particular environment (including the body or a part of the body).

"We depend on a vast army of microbes to stay alive and well: a microbiome that protects us against germs, breaks down food to release energy, and produces vitamins" the combined genetic material of the microorganisms in a particular environment.

"Understanding the microbiome—whether human, animal, and environmental—is as important as the human genome"
Yes, it is that important.

The great news is that whilst Intermittent Fasting we flush out a majority of bad bacteria from our gut, however, as always, it varies from person to person. It has been created by processed foods, chemicals, toxins and many things that can be stored in our gut. If we don't have our microbiome balanced, as well as not feeding the good bacteria to keep it healthy and let it multiply, then we can be in trouble.

There have been 2 studies recently into this

Study 1 – The Influence of the Microbiome on the Metabolism of Diet and Dietary Components

https://www.ncbi.nlm.nih.gov/books/NBK154098/

The main gist of this paper is that it shows that there is growing evidence that gut microbiome influences what your body is able to extract from your diet (what you eat) both energetically and nutritionally.

In effect it tells us that it doesn't really matter how healthily we are eating. If our microbiomes are off balance, then they won't take the food and transform it to the nutrient we need.

(At the time of writing this I have spoken with 2 women in the last week that have tested on the very low side of certain vitamins/minerals: one B12, the other folate acid. They both told me they eat healthy fresh and practically organic diets)

Our microbiomes may have been badly affected by our previous diet and lifestyle. They need to now be fed with foods to benefit them. This study has also shown that obesity correlates with an increase in firmicutes (bad gut bacteria) and a decrease in Bacteroidetes (good gut bacteria). Obesity can sometimes have nothing to do with the food that we eat. How many times do we hear, or have you thought *'I don't really eat that unhealthily, why am I so out of shape?'* - I used to say and think this as do many women I have coached.

We get so stuck with the quality of our food.

It is often the quality of the microbes that is compromised. This can cause weight gain and also stall weight loss in some people.

Bear with me I have a solution after the next study...

Study 2: Gut Microbiota as an Important Modulator of Metabolism, Health and Disease

https://pubs.rsc.org/en/content/articlelanding/2018/ra/c8ra080 94a#!divAbstract

This study mainly tells that microbe diversity of obese individuals is lower than of healthy individuals.

There are thousands of different microbes in the gut. We must eat a diverse range of foods to grow these good healthy microbes (good bacteria). This will then enable the microbiome to work properly and help with absorbing the nutrients we need. It will also affect fat burning in a positive way.

When shopping for fruit and veg, try to go to a fruit and veg store that sells their products loose and select different types of lettuce, tomatoes, potatoes, peas, broccoli. These stores let you fill your basket with whatever you want even if it's just one of each – I do that sometimes and your gut will thank you for that.

I recommend that you feed your microbiome; a diverse range of foods this is what I recommend. Your "diet" (the food you eat each day) should include at least one from the first 2 headings below and a range of the foods from the 3rd heading.

Probiotics – Sauerkraut (unpasteurised), raw kefir, kimchi, kombucha. (Try and have one of these fermented foods or drinks each day.

Prebiotics – Hemp seed, flax seed. chia seeds, sesame seeds (just scatter seeds on everything they are amazing), asparagus, onions.

Polyphenol - Olives, nuts, broccoli. tomatoes, berries, banana, peas and a wide and diverse range of green vegetables

This is just a small example of the diverse range of foods to include in your diet. The sauerkraut (not supermarket bought as they are full of sugar), when I first started eating it, I was not keen at all, I now love it. Just mix it in with your food-mix it into a salad, a stew, or whatever you're having some days. If you can include as much of the above into your diet, then you will be on your way to your microbiome working the way it should.

This particularly applies to women whose weight loss may have stalled or seems slower than everyone else's. However, it is a great idea for everyone as it benefits everyone's overall general health

Chapter 12

Fasting for Health

We are curing ourselves, preventing illness and keeping ourselves well – why isn't everybody fasting?

I often hear women saying, *"Well, I can't help this as it's happened to all the women in my family"*. Now I know that there are cancer genes that are genetic as well as other illnesses, these are real. However, very often illnesses that we think we have inherited from our family are simply down to limiting beliefs – my mother told me I would get it, so I got it! My mother told me all the women in our family put on weight when they hit their forties – I believed it and followed the pattern. Was it true? Yes, because I made it true! It could be as simple as that. In a later chapter I will address limiting beliefs in more detail. For now, just consider that we may be the purveyors of our own illnesses as we have trusted and believed the person that told us we were going to suffer in some sort of way because it ran in our family, or women put on weight in the menopause, or because you're a certain class this happens to us all!

Then there is lifestyle. I have heard women say type 2 diabetes runs in our family! Well, I'm sorry, but type 2 diabetes is not a genetic disease; it is created by lifestyle and food choices. Can it be reversed? Yes, it can. Can you stop your children from getting it? Yes, you can. It's all about diet (meaning what you eat and drink) and lifestyle. This also applies to many other 'modern day' illnesses that attack our immune system and are inflammatory.

We absolutely have to change our relationship with food for ourselves and for our children.

I am so happy to tell you that I have worked with women who have completely turned their health around from many different illnesses with the help of Intermittent Fasting the Life Begins way.

One who sticks out in my mind is Jenny who joined me on a 1/1-month long program. Jenny had had a hell of a year. She had been through more than most of us could bear with part of her family being wiped out in a horrid road traffic accident. Here is Jenny's story in her own words...

"In January 2017 I picked up a virus that landed me in intensive care with lung failure. It transpired that, unbeknown to me, I had been living with COPD (Chronic Obstructive Pulmonary Disorder) for some time. Ironically, I weighed 50kg at the time and was being encouraged to put some weight on by my doctor. I really struggled to put that weight on until randomly, a year later, I started gaining massive amounts, huge amounts of weight! As it turns out I had managed to double my body weight in just 8 weeks. My thyroid gland had gone on strike - just my luck.

Fast forward to January 2020, and my consultant said to me, "You have around 2 years left to live, and I want to put you forward for a double lung transplant, but you need to lose some weight first."

I already knew I was sick; I knew it wasn't great but knowing you're 2 short years from death... there are no words to describe the emotional wreckage. So, I decided to keep that little nugget to myself and battle on trying to lose some weight. The doctor had said that if I made it to 77kg I could start the transplant process. I just needed to lose 10kg and we would take it from there.

I saw one of my Facebook friends had been following an Intermittent Fasting program with Susan and she was having an intake, so I decided to get in contact. I spoke to Susan, and I knew right there and then I had made a life changing decision and I wasn't wrong.

Intermittent Fasting has just slotted into my life with ease. I wasn't one for eating breakfast, so I just had to tackle some niggling eating habits like eating meals at 10pm when my husband got home from work and snacking before he would get in. I now eat with my daughter after school and don't feel the need to snack in the evening before bed.

I still can't get over how much more energy I started to develop very early on in the program. I had a lot more stamina when I am using my home gym. Exercise is crucial but very difficult when you have COPD, but I was finding I could breathe easier.

After 14 weeks of doing Intermittent Fasting, I was finally given the go ahead from my consultant to begin the testing process for my lung transplant as my BMI was now within range. Testing has begun and it's all going really well. I'm not going to curse myself, but I have my fingers crossed. In total, with the huge love and support from all around me, I have now lost 14kg after six months and that's a win, but even bigger for me is my ability to have the stamina to cycle 20k on my exercise bike, to smile and to be kind to myself as I can only do my best.

Susan not only offers advice and information but gives tremendous emotional support and a deep understanding of human emotion."

At the time of writing this book, Jenny has been through testing and is on the transplant list. We hope and pray the right match comes up for her.

There is nothing better than having the energy to go about your day with a smile on your face and no longer feeling like you are walking through treacle. One of my clients who experienced this was Amy, who before joining us was housebound and going through the very of worst of health. Amy joined me last year initially in our 27-day 1/1 program.

Here is her story in her own words…

"I just wanted to share my story for anyone thinking of joining Susan. I started my IF journey on 30th November

2020. I had been diagnosed with Trigeminal Neuralgia the previous year and was on anti-convulsant medication which had contributed to a weight gain, being unable to function at work, unable to exercise, and saw me struggling to enjoy my time with grandchildren. I had brain fog, menopause symptoms etc. I was not in a good place. Following an inspiring 1:1 with Susan, I took the plunge. Fast forward to today and-

♥ *I am off almost all my medication*

♥ *Brain fog has lifted*

♥ *My energy levels have soared*

♥ *I am 39lb lighter*

The group is so supportive, and we have had some fantastic Zoom calls with experts in various fields. Susan is always available to answer any questions or to give some supportive encouragement. I love the fact that for once in my life I am not on a diet, yet the weight is coming off."

And there was Sarah, who went from having to attend her diabetes clinic every month to this…

"Just wanted to share a wee bit about my journey - sorry for the long post.

Today for me is a happy joyful day. I started my journey roughly 6 months ago. 2020 was particularly hard for most of us. For me, way back at beginning of this pandemic, I lost my cousin and my much-loved mother-in-law within a week of each other due to COVID. It was very sudden and under the worst circumstances, a living nightmare. The week of the funeral, my son-in-law lost his job and my daughter's offshore consulting job became non-existent. They suddenly became a young family with 3 kids and no income.

In May I was bed ridden with sciatica and back problems. For a whole week I was unable to get out of bed to the bathroom; what more could life throw at me!! I was just getting back on my feet and twisted my knee- an old injury from previous dislocation flared up and I was walking with 2 sticks. Work was stressful and busy with little or no time to react, due to COVID and panic buying. I would end up lying on my stomach working on a laptop in bed. Then everything crashed and I had a meltdown, not depression but grief, and everything else piled on top with the realisation that I couldn't continue as I was.

I am an extremely strong woman normally, but everything caught up with me. Following a couple of weeks break, I decided I needed to do something. This was when I enrolled on this program with Susan Stewart!! Not primarily to lose weight, but to improve my overall health, my wellbeing, and hopefully get things back under control.

As I said at the beginning, this is a happy day. I have type 2 diabetes and had to attend a clinic regularly for many years. Today my diabetic nurse called with my results. Her conversation started with a surprised question- "What have you been doing?!" My bloods are down from 93 to 54, and cholesterol from 4.5-4.1. She is now suggesting an annual review if this continues. I am eating foods I love- whole foods, no low fat or artificial sweeteners. I love water. If I eat something that doesn't agree with me, I know about it. I have lost 1 1/2 stones. I am not perfect, I lapse, but I don't give myself a hard time. No diet, no guilt, and I love who I am and what I'm doing for the first time in a long time. I am so thankful. I hope this encourages you ladies and you keep on going. Tomorrow is a new day, and the best is yet to come."

These are only 3 stories from the thousands of women I have worked with. A list of ailments that have either become more manageable or even reversed through IF are

- Cancer recovery
- Long COVID
- Fatty liver disease
- Fibromyalgia
- Type 2 diabetes
- Arthritis (I completely cured myself of this)
- Polycystic ovaries
- Cardiovascular problems
- Lung transplant testing
- Gastric problems
- Blood pressure
- Gall bladder problems
- Adrenal fatigue
- Pancreatic episodes
- Menopause
- COVID induced type 2 diabetes

I would like here to address COVID in particular and other viruses that invade our bodies, I am often asked should I continue fasting and my answer is always YES! For these reasons:

- When you are in ketosis, cells are primed to stop viral replication
- At 15 hours fasted, the body will start detoxing bad pathogens – aka autophagy
- Drink bone broth during your eating window as the glycine repairs your gut, where 80% of your immune system lives
- Follow your intuition – it will tell you if fasting is the right thing to do.

Be aware of sugar craving if you have a virus as most– COVID-19 included – propel around your body on blood sugar. The virus is very clever and will make you crave sugars to enable it to spread inwards.

Apart from COVID19, I have not had one day of illness since I started fasting. I have enjoyed the best of health; have great energy levels and I honestly feel like I am in my thirties not my sixties! No more arthritis, no more anxiety, no more brain fog, and no more catching bugs every few weeks.

So, I ask again, why are we not all fasting?

- I believe the obvious answer is Big Pharma doesn't want us to be curing or preventing our illnesses or conditions without their expensive medicines and drugs with all their side effects
- The food industry doesn't want us to eat less
- The diet industry doesn't want us to succeed. Yes, I said it! They rely on 84% of us failing and coming back to them. They need repeat business and rely on us returning. Would it surprise you to know one of the biggest 'diet' companies in the world is owned by a confectionary company!

My darlings, the choice is yours. You can either empower yourself and take control of your health and wellbeing, or hand it over to outside forces.

I am not saying that there isn't a time of place for medicines and drugs. They are vital for some, but if we fast daily and help our body work the way it should then we are well on the way to fantastic health.

You can take this book and work with the information I have shared with you. Start your fasting lifestyle or if you would enjoy my support, I continue to run 1-1 programs and my membership is always open to new members. A community is always helpful when you are on a journey to a new way of life, and it is a beautiful supportive sisterhood full of women who will hold your hand and share their best advice. I am also in their daily to help you on your way to the very best of health, happiness and sustainable weight loss

Chapter 13

Fasting and Mental Health

There are so many 'side effects' from fasting and the effect it has on the way you handle stress. Anxiety and depression are conditions that can see a benefit. I used to be a highly stressed and anxious being. I operated from a *'what will go wrong'* mentality. In some ways it served me well. In my work in the corporate world, I would have plan A, B, C, D right the way through to Z as I would have worked out what could go wrong. I realise now this was my anxiety that caused this.

Now I'm not saying that I am now blasé about all eventualities. I do still think about things going wrong. I do still text my grown children to watch the roads when it's icy, and I do worry if they are away on one of their adventures, but I don't worry as much as I used to.

I know that I now handle stress and anxiety in a different way. For me, IF quells my anxiety because it changes what my mind focuses on. Anxiety is a malfunctioning survival mechanism. Similar to fear, anxiety is designed to help us avoid compromising positions. However, this tool gets its wires crossed and can lead to more discomfort and suffering than it is preventing. It can come in the form of overthinking, but this is not always the case. For me, it sometimes manifests as overthinking, other times it manifests as *over feeling,* where it heightens my emotions. However, when I fast, I notice that neither occur as often. My anxiety is still there, but it is squashed to the point where I can ignore it. Why? For me, it feels like this happens because now my mind is focused on a different type of survival, a more primal type. By reducing my food intake, my mind decides to focus less on general anxieties and instead looks towards the next meal. But I am in a position where I don't need to worry about where my next meal comes from, so this short circuits my anxiety. Leaving it with nowhere to go.

The second possible reason relates, to a process called ketosis, which is where the body runs out of carbohydrates to burn for energy, so instead burns fat and a substance called *ketones,* which are a type of chemical, produced by the liver when insulin levels are low. Ketosis is something that naturally happens during intermittent fasts, as there is no way to fast without running out of carbohydrates.

A study has shown that ketones are effective at managing neurological disorders, as well as symptoms of other disorders such as anxiety. Tests regarding ketone supplementation were performed on several species of rats, where researchers noticed a significant drop in anxiety-related behaviour. While these tests were not replicated on humans, there are anecdotal reports of people finding intermittent fasting to be helpful for their anxiety. I hit ketosis every day and am so happy that it offers me this benefit to my mental health.

Improves memory

Restricting some the hours when you eat has been shown to significantly improve memory, according to a study in the *Journal of the Academy of Nutrition and Dietetics*. In this study, after 4 weeks of Intermittent Fasting, performance on a spatial planning and working memory task, and on a working memory capacity test increased significantly.

Additional research on animals has found that Intermittent Fasting improves learning and memory.

Brightens mood

Research in the *Journal of Nutrition Health & Aging* found that after 3 months of intermittent fasting, study participants reported improved moods and decreased tension, anger, and confusion. Another study from 2018 that was investigating weight-loss strategies, found that intermittent fasting was associated with significant improvements in emotional wellbeing and depression.

There have been many studies on dementia being related to metabolic diseases like hypertension and type 2 diabetes, which is a huge worry. However, these studies have also shown that the relationship between dietary patterns and therapeutic approaches for preventing dementia have been positive.

It has been shown that intermittent fasting reduces DNA damage and inflammatory signalling, can activate and boost plasticity, contributes to and improves the impairment of plasticity within the brain. A few studies have reported dramatic decreases in blood pressure values after intermittent fasting as well as improvement in vascular function. There is also evidence that IF increases insulin sensitivity in neurones and even encourages regrowth of healthy neurones.

Animal studies on Intermittent Fasting have consistently demonstrated disease modifying benefits on a wide range of chronic disorders including obesity, diabetes, cardiovascular disease, cancers, and neurodegenerative diseases. Studies in animals show that Intermittent Fasting enhances cognition in multiple areas of memory and learning.

Intermittent Fasting in animal studies has been shown to reduce brain inflammation. There is strong evidence that forms of Intermittent Fasting can delay the onset and progression of Alzheimer's disease and Parkinson's disease in animal models. Researchers are now exploring opportunities to study Intermittent Fasting in humans; particularly the effect this might have on neurodegenerative diseases, including Alzheimer's disease.

"In animal studies, intermittent fasting has been shown to increase longevity, improve cognitive function and reduce brain plaque as compared with animals fed on a regular diet," said Allan Anderson, MD, Director of the Banner Alzheimer's Institute in Tucson. *"One hypothesis is that intermittent fasting enables cells to remove damaged proteins. It has been shown to delay the onset and progression of disease in animal models of Alzheimer's disease and Parkinson's."*

Leading experts in this field of study have been researching Intermittent Fasting for many years. Our bodies predominantly use glucose produced by the food we eat for fuel. But when we fast, the body turns to alternate energy sources including fat. Fat metabolism leads to the production of ketone bodies which have been linked to improved thinking, learning and memory in animal studies.

In a review of Intermittent Fasting research in the December 2019 issue of the *New England Journal of Medicine*, the technique showed promise in animal models for a wide range of chronic disorders. The authors' conclusion was that calorie restriction in animals increases life span, improves cognition and can even reverse the effects of obesity, diabetes and brain inflammation.

I often say that Intermittent Fasting gets your happy on literally and there is so much proof now that it does.

Chapter 14

Enjoying Your New Way of Life

Will I fast forever? Yes, I will, I couldn't bear not to feel as good as I feel now. If I stop for any length of time, I need to get back to it as soon as I return from holiday, the wedding, or event I have attended is over. My joints start to ache, I feel bloated, tired, and not mentally alert. It doesn't take long to feel like that. This is the beauty of a lifestyle change. You just have to get back to it as you know you feel SOOOO good.

You will be exactly the same – it really is a lifestyle change. After your first 3 to 4 months, your foundations will have been built. You are a faster and your body recognises that you are a faster. Never worry if you have a holiday or a sociable weekend- there is no 'wagon' to fall off, you won't have 'blown it'. In fact, please enjoy your life and know that you will get straight back to your fasting.

You will live a life of health and happiness, and you will reach a weight and size that your body decides is right for you. I have gone down to a size 12 sometimes a size 14 (UK sizes). Yeah, I know sizes aren't generalised anymore. In fact, some brands will purposely size their clothes to a smaller size number to make you feel good.

What will really make you feel good is noticing your:

- energy rising and being constant,
- your skin glowing,
- your aches and pains leaving you,
- inflammatory diseases diminishing as a benefit of fasting,
- You will find YOU again. That feeling is awesome! It's like a little whisper at first- *"Oh, there I am"*. It feels familiar and, as time goes on, you realise this is the way we are meant to feel: free, fit, healthy and happy.

As your fasting lifestyle goes on, you will find that you don't have to rely on clocks and schedules. You will hear your body when you are actually hungry, and you will then open your eating window. You will know when you have finished eating for the day and are totally satisfied. A top tip at this point is to brush your teeth when you close your eating window– it will be a signal to you that you are now in your fasting window. It is also good to mix it up a bit, by not sticking rigidly to the same times each day and by listening to your body you will achieve this.

Water is always vital, and you should now be past having to measure it. The minimum of 2.5 litres when fasting is simply a rough guide, you will go into your own flow and probably drink a lot more. Water is now my drink of choice all day long and I always have a bottle beside me. I now drink out of a lovely glass bottle with a rose quartz crystal in it. This is my choice and wouldn't suit everyone, I just love crystals so it's the right vessel for me. When I started fasting, I used to drink a bottled mineral water as I had read that this was good for fasting however, I realised that I was probably simply buying plastic bottles and my recycling bin would fill up. I quickly became happy with tap water. You can buy a water filter jug if you would like to.

The vessel that you drink your water from is important. It needs to be something you enjoy drinking from and that is down to your personal choice. I have gone from crystal glasses to aluminium cooling bottle to a plastic bottle with a straw and now onto my bottle with my rose quartz crystal. I'm sure I will find something else I like in the future and change again! Your enjoyment of your water is vital to the fasting process so make it as easy and enjoyable as you can.

When I hear people say, *"Yeah, I'm fasting but just not drinking water as much as I should"*– I have to tell them that they're not fasting! I have covered previously why this is, but your water is vital to enable your body to go into all the beautiful benefits that fasting offers you. If you're not drinking the water then your body thinks you're dieting and won't go into autophagy, human growth hormone or ketosis. In fact, it will hang onto the fat cells as it will be wondering what you are going to do next.

What about holidays and socialising?

The flip side of Intermittent Fasting is wonderful intermittent feasting. When you save all your fuel for the day to eat in a shorter time period, you get to eat pretty luxuriously during that time every single day. This makes Intermittent Fasting (IF) perfect for the holiday season. If you haven't intermittently fasted through a holiday before, you might be wondering how you're going to handle the questions people will ask you about your new way of eating and whether you'll have to skip brunch with friends to stay on schedule. Practicing IF through a holiday season and having brunch with your friends is definitely achievable. It can be freeing if you go into it with a plan. Here are some tips for how to talk about IF (or not), what to do when someone nice brings you a cookie, whether or not to take a day off, and how to get back on track when you do.

What to tell people

Plan A: Nothing.

Most of the time, you actually don't have to talk about it. It's usually simple to add an hour or two to your fast or extend your eating window a bit so that parties fall within the time that you plan to eat. In this case, you just fast most of the day, eat something festive with friends or family, and close your eating window. Nothing out of the ordinary there for people to ask you about. If the event just isn't going to fit into your eating window—or if the food isn't worth opening your window for—you still may not need to talk about it. You can get some water or black coffee and focus on the people you came to see.

Most people aren't monitoring what you eat and won't notice if you don't.

Plan B: If someone does notice, you can tell them you ate earlier (yesterday is earlier) or that you have plans to eat later (because you do). That's enough to handle a lot of situations.

Plan C: If your friend or loved one is nosier or not satisfied by that explanation, go ahead and explain that you're doing IF and your eating window opens later (or closed earlier). Hopefully, they'll be interested and supportive. If they're not, I'm sorry. Don't worry, though. There's plenty of research to help you stand up for yourself. If they're worried that you're crashing your metabolism by not eating, you can point them to this study that shows short-term fasting (between 12 and 72 hours) actually increases metabolic rate. You might be well-adjusted to fat-burning, feeling amazing, and seeing results. Mention that. There's nothing like results to convince these sceptics.

If you're just starting your IF lifestyle and are still in the adjustment phase, you probably won't have results to talk about yet. In that case, you can point out that everyone actually eats on a schedule. No one eats 24/7 except for infants, and their main goal in life is to gain weight. The schedule you were following before didn't work for you and your life, so you're trying a new one.

Whether or not to take a day off?

I'm a firm believer that the way you eat should support your life; your life should not be spent supporting the way you eat. You have better things to do. Family, friends, and celebrations are some of the things that make life wonderful. Want to have breakfast with a friend who's only in town once a year? Go for it! Please let the people in your life be more important than food. Going to a celebration at midnight after your window is normally closed? It's ok to enjoy it. Eat, drink, and be merry. Make a memory. This is your life. If it's truly a once-a-year thing, or a friend you're not able to see often, it can be a good choice to indulge. You'll have to weigh that against what your goals are, how fast you want to reach them, and the way you'll feel the next day.

Here's why taking a day off can affect how you feel the next day. IF works because after you're adjusted to it, you use up your glycogen stores every day and switch to burning fat for fuel. When you refill your glycogen stores so much that you're not able to use them all up during your next fast, it's only one fast, you will quickly re-adjust and get straight back to fat burning the next day. You could feel hungry or sluggish as you get back into your normal IF rhythm, but that will return really quickly. Is it worth it? Sometimes. Some people really don't like the way they feel after eating all day, so they choose a longer 8- to 10-hour window on special occasions instead of a complete day off. If you're just starting, though, an eight-hour window might not feel that long to you. That's ok. You're free to do what you need to in order to make IF support your life.

If I'm having a night out, I will do a longer fast, and I will slip my eating window forward by 2 sometimes 4 hours depending in the night out planned, i.e., if I normally open my window at 12, I will move it forward and open it at 2pm or 4pm. I will use a couple of grains of pink Himalayan salt to keep me going and keep busy. Then, the next day, I just open my eating window as normal. In the festive period I usually have a Christmas Day and a Boxing Day fasting 12/14 hours a day, by the day after Boxing Day I cannot wait to get back to my schedule. I've had a fab time and probably feel a bit sluggish and bloated. It usually subsides within a couple of days back on my 18-hour fasting.

Try not to feel guilty. Life is different every day and that's not a bad thing. Close your window when you're ready on your beautifully indulgent day. You may take a shorter-than-usual fast the next day and eat during your normal window. That's it. You're back on schedule. If you have low energy or feel hungry the next day or two, use more water, extra naps, or one or two low-carb meals... sorted! This mini adjustment after a day or 2 off is typically not as difficult or as long as your initial adapting to fasting. You can do it. Make IF fit your life. IF can be an amazing way to maintain or possibly even lose weight during a season when both are more challenging than usual. Allow yourself to have a holiday. Follow your own schedule–or don't. Enjoy your friends, family, and food to the max. If your times get skewed one day, just fix them the next and keep going. It's your life, and you can adjust the way you eat until it works for you. You don't have to worry or feel guilt for the way you eat–especially during celebrations. MOST OF ALL, HAVE THE VERY BEST GUILT FREE FESTIVE OR HOLIDAY SEASON!

You may find that after holiday seasons you find that sugar has crept back into your eating and you may be feeling lethargic, inflammation may have set in, and your brain might go a bit foggy. This is the time to do another liver cleanse previously mentioned and detailed at the back of the book. This will regulate you, trigger your liver to work perfectly as the filter it is, and change your tastebuds back to saying NO to sugar most of the time.

Will you never eat sugar again? Of course, you will. The difference now, is that probably 8/10 times you will make the choice to say NO, happily! Those 2 other times make sure that you enjoy whatever you have decided to eat, eat it slowly, mindfully, enjoying every morsel and feel good that you've had it. Life is for living!

The same philosophy applies with alcohol. I know I have mentioned it before, but I will say it again- when you choose to have a little drink, savour it, sip it, take it slowly, and enjoy it's effect. You will naturally then drink less of it.

Rest assured that the rest of your life will be the best of your life. A life full of energy, wearing clothes you're comfortable in, and knowing that you are doing the very best for your health and longevity.

I used to think I would die young! Why? Because I thought I was hopeless, a lost cause, so unhealthy and I could never get a hold of my health because I failed at every diet I ever did. I would tell myself I had an addictive personality which was inherited from my dad! He had been an alcoholic at one time in his life – a Martini alcoholic – yes, he was such a different man. He hasn't had a drink for decades. I thought my eating and sometimes drinking habits were in my genes!

I no longer believe I will die young. I believe I am going to live a long, healthy, active, energised life. I feel 30 years you longer than I did 5 years ago, and I look 20 years younger too! I say that from a place of love not ego. I thank myself every day for the kindness and love I give my body.

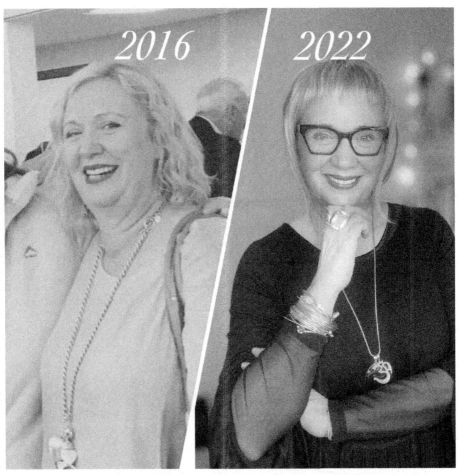

We can talk ourselves in and out of things so easily but these beliefs that limit us, are they excuses? Maybe! There is a limiting beliefs exercise at the back of the book. I encourage you to do it, it will quickly free you from these things that we believe are part of us!

You will go on and live your life completely in control of your own beautiful body- what you nourish it with, and how often you cleanse. It is such a beautiful and freeing feeling. It is true that the body freedom you obtain and the ripple effects throughout your life are immense.

- You learn patience,
- your self-esteem rises,
- you become powerful because you know that if you've done this you can do anything!
- You learn to say no with grace.
- Your relationships blossom
- Your life truly begins

I want every woman and man to feel this!

Testimonials

There are so many reasons to introduce Intermittent Fasting into your life and I have covered some of them in this book. I believe the world should be living this way and we would cure so many ills. We would be able to help keep ourselves well and live long and healthy lives. This is my wish for you and all of mankind.

I couldn't imagine living in a different way. The reassurance that I am keeping myself well and doing the very best I can to be the Best Version of Me keeps me secure and happy. The ripple effects through my life have been immense, from running after my grandkids to complete self-belief that I can do whatever I set my mind too.

Add to that, the women that I have coached over the past few years who are living their best life, cured their ills and are FREE from food guilt and diets forever

Here are some of their testimonials in their own words.

Mary testimonial

Intermittent Fasting has changed my life, quite literally.

I have never been a dieter or followed dietary plans. I have always advocated the drinking of water, so this was also a habit I had got into.

I have always preferred to eat less and more sensibly and actively participate in outdoors pursuits. I have always loved fresh fruit and vegetables and have always included these in my meal preparations. I also prefer to always prepare fresh daily meals.

Why did I start the plan?

When reading Susan's claims about IF I realised this was for me.

- *I had put on a bit of weight during the pandemic: the heaviest ever!*

- *Lockdown was restricting my daily ability to move naturally.*
- *My clothes had become tight but still fitted me – just!*
- *My gut was not functioning as it should.*
- *I was always hungry!*
- *I had health issues...*
- *I realised that fasting would support me in my goals to not only lose weight but, as a side effect, my constant feeling of being hungry might be caseated.*
- *My bowel was causing me great issues during lockdown.*
- *I also regularly looked 7 months pregnant and resorted to buying a pair of pregnancy tights!*

8 months later....

- *I find my fasting hours suit me*
- *My hunger craving has gone*
- ***I have lost over 2 stones – 32lbs***
- *I enjoy all the water I drink*
- *I enjoy all the things I used to love but in moderation*
- *Sugar is not in my diet*

• I have followed Susan's monthly guidelines and slowly it became easier and easier to keep to the fasting hours that I set to exclude breakfast and give me a late lunch and early supper. I continued to drink plenty of water and enjoy black coffee and green tea. I no longer have sugar cravings.

• I love my ability to eat when hungry and to enjoy anything I want

• This IF eating regime will be my saviour for the rest of my life and will hopefully prevent very invasive surgery. It has become a very easy way of life.

Stephanie's story

It was Susan that inspired me, watching her info videos on Instagram. I really felt down about myself, and I listened and thought this is my chance to change myself and my lifestyle
The first two weeks were a challenge, but my determination got me through that and then it became a way of life, and I have never found it a challenge since.

My hair and skin are much healthier. I feel fit, and I have started to have faith in myself. The Program fitted into my daily routines with no problems at all

My favourite part has been buying clothes that don't fit and then getting into them. That feeling is amazing! I have only weighed myself twice. I find this is better for me and I get to buy something new! I am 2 sizes smaller already.

I would recommend this to anyone having tried all sorts of diets. I would say don't do them- this is the way to change your life, gain better health and enjoy being yourself.

Dierdre's story

A big thank you to you Susan! I am in such a better place as this year comes to a close. I spent 2021 focusing on becoming my best me.

First, I worked to heal old traumas, then found my place of power and discovered my zone of genius. After so much internal soul work, I knew that the natural next step was to work on healing my body.

So began my IF journey. And what a journey it's been with COVID thrown into the mix. But now I am in control of my food, my water and for the first time in ten years I feel comfortable in the skin that I'm in.

Not shrinking back or hiding. Free to be me. Blessed from the inside out. Just wanted to let you know personally just how much that means to me.

I am a size 12 for the first time since my teens and I feel amazing.

These changes have rippled outwards to improve my relationships with my children, my husband, our marriage, our family, my friendships and the people that I meet. Deep thanks from the bottom of my heart.

Ann's story

After researching what IF was, I had planned to start it "sometime"

.

By perfect timing I saw a post by Susan Stewart about how she mentors' women on their journey to start and establish IF. After messaging Susan and filling out an application form, I was accepted onto my initial 6-month journey with an established group of female intermittent fasters.

The experience has been great.

Susan is unbelievable in supporting your journey. She is there every step of the way and has a vast amount of knowledge in the area. Anything she is not sure about she will find out for you from her own team of mentors, including an internationally renowned IF specialist who is a doctor.

The Facebook group is very supportive the women. They are encouraging and share their own experiences, tips, hints and tricks for the most positive outcomes. Included in the community is access to experts in holistic skincare, personal trainer and a spiritual specialist who are regular contributors. As well as guest experts who come on monthly live for Zoom calls. There are weekly live Zooms where you can ask anything and seek support in all areas of the program.

IF is amazing for the body, it helps the body heal and regenerate on a daily basis. Every day that you fast your body deep cleanses and gets rid of toxic cells and replaces them with healthy cells (autophagy); human growth hormone kicks in and is anti-ageing. It also aids in helping you to look after your bones, muscles and your metabolic rate as well as going into fat and glycogen burn.

I have embedded "Life Begins" fasting into my life and will continue forever.

Eileen testimonial

Earlier this year, I developed a shoulder injury which caused me incredible pain. I was unable to do many things, even little stuff, like getting dressed, filling the kettle, drying my hair... all things you do without thinking, became unbelievably difficult to do and achieving any of them would hurt so much and take me ages. I couldn't even go out for a walk without hurting, so I became very withdrawn and introspective. I was so tired but dreaded going to bed, because I hurt so much, and I couldn't sleep. I'd been prescribed painkillers, but they upset my stomach so much (the stomach pain was worse than the shoulder pain) ... it was horrendous. This was all during lockdown, so I was unable to see family either, and essentially I was in a very dark place.

I had to do something to change what was going on and conventional medicine obviously wasn't helping. So, having previously read about what Susan was doing with Intermittent Fasting, I thought I would give it a go. I hummed and hawed about it for ages; I think fear of failure held me back for a while, but by June I'd decided enough was enough! Susan had 27 days offer on, so I signed up for it, thinking I could at least manage that long. We had a good chat and she advised on coping strategies which I found helpful.

After just a few days on the program, I found that the pain I'd been having was lessening and I was finally able to sleep well. My energy levels increased over the next couple of weeks and by the end of the 27 days, I was almost a different person. I've carried on with the IF and find my skin is clearer, my cellulite has smoothed out and is almost gone! It hadn't particularly bothered me before, but this was a benefit

I hadn't expected! However, the best thing for me (apart from losing a few unwanted pounds) was that the inflammation which had been causing my shoulder pain had disappeared! I still have stiffness, but that's improving daily. I'm in awe of how my body has been able to heal itself in just a couple of months. I look forward to every day now and am enjoying life again, and it's all thanks to joining Susan's programme. I'd advise anyone who is in two minds, as I was, to give it a go.

Linda's Story

I just wanted to share my intermittent fasting journey with you all.

After recovering from COVID last year, I was left with food allergies that I never had before, so I tried a food diary and elimination for many months. I cut out dairy, all processed foods (not that I ate many) and ate mostly organic. It worked to a point, and I had been watching Susan's weight loss and health journey with interest.

So, I joined her fabulous 1 to 1 program on the 1st of April and have been on my fasting journey since then. I don't eat breakfast anyway, so I found it easy to get started. I have lost just under a stone in weight, and I found a waist I didn't know I had! My skin is glowing, my bingo wings have disappeared, my allergies are under control, and I am hydrated and feeling fabulous.

I have re-set my immune system as it were, and this will be my eating plan for the rest of my life. I can honestly say it wasn't hard, apart from the water drinking because I wasn't used to it, but I have not cheated or deviated from the wonderful advice given to be by Susan Stewart and she knows her stuff. If anyone is still unsure if it's for them, just give it a go, your body and mind will thank you.

Update –6 months later, Linda's allergies have completely left her, she is a size 10 for the first time since her teenage years and feels so amazing – like a teenager she says!

Mary's story

Susan is a lovely ray of light and has been so supportive and inspiring! I joined the fast-track program after reading a great review from a friend. After being unwell recently, I was keen to boost my immune system and feel better about myself with some weight loss.

I had fallen into bad eating habits. I lacked energy, felt awful and through the program was able to identify that I did not ever drink water!?

I am now recognising that drinking water and listening to my body makes me feel good! I never expected to have an increase in energy and clarity so quickly. I am enjoying now feeling no bloating in the evenings and surprisingly don't crave the snacks like I used to anymore. Thank you, Susan!

Michelle - my story so far....

November began with me feeling pretty hopeless and with the usual feeling of 'I must start to toe the line in January'. Anyhow, I was on Facebook and randomly saw a post of Susan's. This well-spoken, glowing, shiny lady talking about something that could transform our lives. I was interested but sceptical, as I have honestly been on every diet known to woman!! Anyway, I listened and thought...this is something I think I could do.

I spoke to Susan who talked me through the program, and it sounded great.

I took to it quite well...with encouragement from the group and Zoom calls. Within a couple of days...yes, as quick as that...I started to feel better in myself. Not weight loss yet, but I am not bloated now. I feel a bit lighter in myself somehow. I am sleeping better too.

Fast forward to just before Christmas, I was 7lbs lighter and I felt amazing. More confident that this was something I could sustain.

Thank you, Susan, for your consistent encouragement!

Some Helpful Information and Exercises

on Limiting Beliefs and Mindset

Limiting Beliefs

In our Life Begins Programs, we introduce Intermittent Fasting as a Lifestyle, and we work with your mind and soul. We can be held back by Limiting Beliefs that really do not serve us in our lives. These can be so deep rooted in our psyche that, no matter what lifestyle change we do, we won't achieve it completely as we are literally limited by these beliefs.

They can be about body confidence; breakfast being the most important meal of the day (after all Granny told us that, didn't she?); you are just 'big boned', the menopause makes you put on weight; all the women in your family start gaining weight in their 30's, it's genetic; when you 'let yourself go' there's no going back; you're not worthy feeling good…this list is endless.

Here are a couple of exercises that are part of the Mind and Soul Section of my website on Limiting Beliefs. Give it a go – it really is so freeing.

I know that I had many Limiting Beliefs which I carried around as baggage for my whole life. Many related to my weight and body image. I remember my Mum telling me when I was in my mid 30's that I looked lovely but, *"Just wait Susan, when you hit 40 you will start putting on weight. I did, your Granny did and look at all your Aunties."*

I know she didn't deliberately or purposefully intend to harm me saying this, but this belief embedded within me and, guess what? At 37 I started gaining weight and started the first of many visits to a slimming club. I now believe that this weight gain wasn't my genetics, but it was a belief that was instilled within me that would then inevitably happen.

The Mind-Body connection is one of the most powerful that we have and if we can deal with this we are on our way to **self-love**, **self-belief** and **freedom!**

What is a Belief?

It's a feeling of certainty about what something means. Beliefs create the maps that guide us toward our goals and give us the power to take action.

The challenge is that most of our beliefs are generalisations about our past, based on our interpretations of painful and pleasurable experiences. Often, we are unconscious about what we believe and how those beliefs affect our actions.

Our limiting beliefs can cause us to miss out on the things that we want most. Our empowering beliefs can drive us toward to the life we want to live.

What is a goal that you have always wanted to achieve and haven't?

Why haven't you?

Whatever your reason, there's always a limiting belief.

Time to Explore!

Think about these questions and journal your answers on the following page.

- What is my current body image?

- How positive do I feel about myself when I look in the mirror?

It's ok to have things you want to change, like get in shape, lose weight, etc. But if you feel a lack of self-worth or extreme feelings about yourself as a person, that is something to take note of. Believe it or not, these feelings can change no matter what your weight is.

- What are your limiting beliefs?

- When was the first time you felt this?

Limiting Beliefs Exercise 2

This may take you a while to do, and it is a good idea to do it over a few days. Write down your limiting beliefs relating to your weight/body in the box below. Think about the first time you felt this, what had happened, who had said it to you, and where were you. Go into as much detail as you can

When you think you have listed them all, visualise yourself putting them one by one in a case. Then, take the case up beside you, open it and take them out one by one and hand the belief back to the person/situation that gave it to you. Sometimes it may be something you told yourself!

Say, *"Thank you for this can you now please take it back, it's not true and no longer serves me."*

Mindset

Next let's consider mindset. There are so many conflicting views on mindset out there from so many schools of thought on mindset being

- Goal-setting mindset.
- Patient mindset.
- Courageous mindset.

- Focused mindset.

- Positive mindset.

- Learning mindset
- Growth mindset
- Abundance mindset

It has been described as complicated and complex and taking a lifetime to learn. I'm not waiting until I'm 80 years old to get this right, and I hope you're not either!

The wonderful **Marissa Peer** in her teachings tells us mindset is as simple as the dialogue that we have with ourselves. The things we say inside our head.

I used to call myself a Stupid Idiot 10 times a day!! Did that serve me well? No. Would I speak to my best friend or daughter like that? No. We can be so cruel to ourselves with this internal dialogue, but we can change it and in turn change our body chemistry and even the cells within our body by being kind to ourselves.

Dr David Hamilton tells us that scientific evidence has proven that being kind to ourselves changes the brain, impacts the heart and immune system, and may even be an antidote to depression.

We're actually genetically wired to be kind. We have to include ourselves in this kindness.

When we're kind, our bodies are healthiest.

At first it may feel unfamiliar and strange, but there are little things you can do to make it work.

When was the last time you told yourself *"I love you?"* I know I had never done so. A lovely easy exercise is when you are brushing your teeth, look yourself in the eye and say in your head '*I Love you*' 10 times. Do it every day. Make it a habit even if you don't believe it at first. Your brain doesn't know the difference between imagination and reality. You will become comfortable doing it and you will feel the difference in your being.

Another way to counteract negative dialogue with ourselves is to speak to ourselves in third person. You can become your own inner coach. In fact, you ARE your own inner coach.

I love Suzy Greaves advice in her book *Making the Big Leap*

    When you're afraid, what does your inner coach say?

    When you feel you're not good enough, what does your inner coach say?

    When you feel ugly, what does your inner coach say?

    When you feel sad, what does your inner coach say?

    When you're tired, what does your inner coach say?

    What script would you have to hear to create the life you really want?

Current Self-dialogue	Positive Self-dialogue
E.g., I'm a stupid idiot	E.g., You made the wrong choice there and thankfully, you are……
E.g., I'm hopeless	E.g., You are amazing; you can make the right choices.

How can you change your self-dialogue?

Write a list below of things you find yourself saying to yourself this month and offer yourself a positive alternative. What would your inner coach say?

When we can get our limiting beliefs and mindset right, everything else will flow. When you rid yourself of beliefs that very often aren't your own, you will fly. When you change your mindset and that internal dialogue that is cruel and doesn't fulfil any purpose apart from holding you back, you will learn to love yourself.

Life Begins is about the complete package- changing your Lifestyle, your Mind and nurturing your soul. It's time to get started and allow your life to truly begin.

5 Day Liver Cleanse

So many of the things we did in our lifestyles over the years will have damaged our liver, and this can often be the core root problem when our fat burning is being stubborn. This is because we could have damaged the functions of our liver, often unknowingly and often not purposefully.

So many toxins affect our liver, from alcohol to living in a damp house. It is good for us all to cleanse our liver from time to time.

Studies show that a high fructose diet is worse for liver damage than calories. Corn syrup, cakes, sweeties, processed foods, juices, diet drinks, salad dressings, sweetened yogurts, high processed fats, cereals and bad oils to name a few. Alcohol also shuts down the fat burn as your liver priorities the alcohol stores it as glycogen and will burn it first before it considers fat burn.

As always, I'm not saying to never eat or drink these things; occasional mindful indulgence is fine.

Let's give our livers a break and a boost by a 5-day cleanse. This could be done regularly, maybe every 6 weeks. These foods can also be incorporated in your diet to help keep your liver working to its best, but let's start with baby steps. Avoid processed foods and refined sugars for 5 days – yes you can do it!

Start with a Castor Oil Pack

Do one at the start of the week on whatever evening suits, before you start the cleanse, and then one at the end of the 5 days.

Leave the pack across your liver for a full 2 hours. It's a good idea to put some sort of plastic – cling film – over it to and a hot water bottle on top of it to retain the heat. Enjoy the 2-hour rest. This will help drain your liver and improve your lymphatic flow.

You can make and use your own castor oil packs with a few materials. Naturopath practitioners recommend looking for hexane-free castor oil. Or you can order one from here is you are in the UK https://shop.herbs-hands-healing.co.uk/product/cold-pressed-castor-oil-pack-kit - but disregard their instructions as they don't pertain to our liver cleanse and are generalised, please follow instructions below.

Ingredients and supplies

To make your own, you'll need these items:

o castor oil – organic

o unbleached wool or cotton flannel – towelling is fine too

o medium container or bowl

o tongs

o scissors

o plastic sheeting, such as a small tablecloth or garbage bag

Directions

1. Cut the wool or cotton flannel into rectangular pieces, about 12 inches by 10 inches.
2. Use at least three to four pieces of cloth to make a pack.
3. Heat the oil to warm. Disclaimer – be careful that you don't let it get too hot. Use around 1/3 of a bottle of castor oil

4. Place over your liver. Place some plastic or cling film over the top and then a hot water bottle
5. Lie down and relax for 2 hours
6. When you remove the pack, just rub the castor oil into your body
7. You can store this pack in an airtight container in the fridge for the next time and simply reheat

Increase Folate and vitamin B12 foods and don't eat and processed foods or refined sugars

Folate foods
o   Leafy Green Veg
o   Citrus Fruits
o   Dry beans
o   Asparagus
o   Beetroot
o   Brussel Sprouts
o   Broccoli
o   Nuts and Seeds
o   Avocado
o   Beans

Vitamin B12 foods

o   Grass Fed Meats
o   Fish
o   Poultry
o   Eggs

Incorporate as many for these in your diet or even be brave and eat only these for 5 days. Try your very best not to eat any processed foods during this time, with no alcohol and no refined sugars

So, you can go on and take all the information in this book, and if you would like my help to take it deeper or for accountability or an absolute personalised plan and coaching you will find me on-

Facebook   -
https://www.facebook.com/groups/intermittentfastthenatural way
Instagram - https://www.instagram.com/iamsusanstewart/
Website – www.intermittentfast.co.uk

I will always support you whether in my free groups or as your coach. I hope you go on and change your life and please share on social media how you get on. Fast On darlings – and Ditch Diets forever.

Printed in Great Britain
by Amazon